Elbow Arthroscopy

Luigi Adriano Pederzini
Gregory Bain · Marc R. Safran

Editors

Elbow Arthroscopy

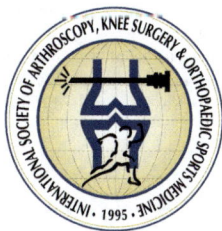

INTERNATIONAL SOCIETY OF ARTHROSCOPY, KNEE SURGERY & ORTHOPAEDIC SPORTS MEDICINE · 1995 ·

Springer

Editors
Luigi Adriano Pederzini
Department of Orthopaedic
   and Arthroscopic
Nuovo Ospedale di Sassuolo
Sassuolo
Italy

Marc R. Safran
Stanford University
Redwood City, CA
USA

Gregory Bain
North Adelaide
Australia

ISBN 978-3-642-38102-7   ISBN 978-3-642-38103-4   (eBook)
DOI 10.1007/978-3-642-38103-4
Springer Heidelberg New York Dordrecht London

Library of Congress Control Number: 2013937197

Printed on acid-free paper

Springer is part of Springer Science+Business Media (www.springer.com)

Foreword

Access to medical education, where basic sciences together with medical innovations and applied technology are needful, represents a challenge of which we are aware and strive to provide worldwide. In order to become reachable, a strong-minded leadership, representative of the five continents, is promoting a unique alliance with national, continental, and specialty societies. *ISAKOS Global Connection* is a project worthy to compromise with, a Campaign for Education, Research, and Collaboration. This is intended to leverage and leveling of the education playing field for arthroscopy, knee surgery, and orthopedic sports medicine around the world.

Both accesses to technology and education technologies are essential to provide equal opportunities. Uneven realities described and emphasized by fellows and residents, arriving from all around the world, along with their extraordinary learning skills and strong motivation, made us realize that ISAKOS and partners have the responsibility to provide an educational umbrella in which all agents would collaborate and profit. Once assumed as our major goal, it is today an admirable ongoing reality. Therefore, one effort supported by many, can bring you into high-performing educational sets, regardless of the zip code you live in. We will join you and you will be joining us in this priceless educational mission. Consequently, allowing you to train with the most advanced techniques with ultimate technologies and under guidance of globally renowned experts. This is the way to assure that high-quality patient care is achieved.

In the subsequent pages of this booklet dedicated to elbow arthroscopy, the reader will be able to get acquainted with the state of the art on that subject. This outstanding and generous share of knowledge conveys a comprehensive resource to education on elbow arthroscopy. It is a secure value and an important reflex of authors' commitment to the educational mission of ISAKOS. The reading you are about to begin, consubstantiates a text from the best to all that have the drive to catch up, and the intrinsic responsibility to provide the best health care to their patients. Science and skills brought to you by this book's authors arises from talented and passionate personalities that bring orthopedics its nobility. ISAKOS Global Connection and Education strives to give no less.

João Espregueira-Mendes
Chairman of the Education Committee

Introduction

The elbow is one of the most complex joints in the body and is surrounded by important neurovascular structures and ligamentous connections. Elbow arthroscopy is a technically demanding surgical procedure that requires precise knowledge of elbow anatomy in various positions, and extensive arthroscopic experience to cope with the limitations. The technique carries greater neurovascular risk and technical challenge than knee or shoulder arthroscopy. However, with a thorough understanding of the anatomy, elbow arthroscopy can provide an opportunity for safe diagnostic and therapeutic intervention in intra- and periarticular pathologies with little morbidity when performed with sound clinical judgment, accurate surgical technique, and appropriate postoperative rehabilitation.

The ISAKOS Elbow Arthroscopy Booklet provides a comprehensive approach to deal with the most common intra- and periarticular elbow pathologies in our daily practice. The booklet begins with the comprehensive description of elbow anatomy, portal replacement, patient setup, and arthroscopic techniques.

Indications for elbow arthroscopy including osteochondritis dissecans, stiff elbow, epicondylitis, instability, and fractures are described in detail. Endoscopy around the elbow and the future of elbow arthroscopy are addressed and allow us to see where the leaders in elbow arthroscopy are using this technology in new and imaginative ways. It is our expectation that this booklet will allow elbow surgeons, who are willing take the time to master the basics, to make decisions that will safely help their patients remain active.

We thank the contributing authors for their work and commitment to present their combined experience in this very valuable and extraordinary text.

Dr. Cüneyt 'John' Tamam
Dr. Gary Poehling

Preface

The development of Elbow Arthroscopy and the advances in technique have evolved as the result of many contributions by surgeons over the last 15 years. Many years before, Burman in the 1930s first affirmed that the elbow joint was nearly impossible to be explored arthroscopically and eventually only the anterior compartment could be examined. In the last several years, academic surgeons in North American reported technical advances that evolved this procedure from being a highly demanding and not so frequent procedure, to one that can now be used with confidence by appropriately trained surgeons. Surgeons focusing on upper limb disorders, approaching the elbow from the shoulder or wrist perspective, reported studies introducing arthroscopic anatomy, portals, and surgical arthroscopic approaches to several elbow pathologies.

First of all, it is necessary to know the anatomy, particularly the periarticular neural and vascular structures, and their relative relationship to the joint and portals, to minimize risk of possible complications. This is particularly important, due to close proximity of the major nerves. In fact, the initial reports of elbow arthroscopy indicated an excessive risk of neurological and vascular complications. As safer techniques were introduced, the prevalence of complications decreased. The great work of these pioneers dedicated to the advancement of elbow arthroscopy has allowed young surgeons to perform this procedure following thorough guidelines and avoiding risks.

The International Society for Arthroscopy Knee Surgery and Orthopaedic Sport Medicine (ISAKOS) several years ago produced an Arthroscopic Atlas of several joints, including the elbow, and then completed a Standard Terminology Project in order to allow surgeons from all over the world to have the same guidelines and the same language in practicing and reporting elbow arthroscopy surgeries.

The Education Committee of ISAKOS charged us, Luigi Pederzini, Marc Safran and Greg Bain, to describe the basic techniques, as well as the more advanced aspects of elbow arthroscopy to allow surgeons to follow the same safe guidelines and to better understand simple and more difficult procedures. The authors who are involved in this project, humbly, have been considered by some to be experts and pioneers of elbow arthroscopy, providing a perspective of elbow arthroscopy from North America, Australia, and Europe. As the reader, you will find these papers of extremely high quality, and may convey the high level of the authors' work and their ability to teach complex procedures in a simple way.

Anatomy is thoroughly introduced referencing safe portals and methods to avoid risk of associated neurovascular complications. Arthroscopic technique is a chapter that provides the anatomy, including portal anatomy, and tips and techniques to perform safe elbow arthroscopy. Further, this chapter serves as a platform on which the more complex concepts are built and described in the following chapters. The chapter on osteochondritis dissecans (OCD) gives an in-depth and detailed description to diagnose and treat this pathology, which occurs frequently in young athletes with as yet still unclear natural history and long-term outcomes. Still connected to sport activity but also to heavy manual workers, epicondylitis is exhaustively presented explaining meticulous techniques and encouraging results. Elbow stiffness remains a common complication after conservative or surgical treatment of elbow pathologies.

This chapter assists the surgeon in describing the causes of stiffness and provides indications for when and how to treat these cases arthroscopically. It also outlines the limitations of arthroscopy and directs the surgeon on when to revert to open surgery in the more complex cases. Arthroscopic treatment of elbow fractures and the future of elbow arthroscopy provides a window into the future, opens new horizons and challenges for elbow surgery. Complications in elbow arthroscopy is one of the most important chapters in this book and the authors provide a review of the milestones in our learning curve and suggest how to avoid these negative results.

This book assists the developing surgeon to be able to perform elbow arthroscopic surgery. For the experienced surgeon, it is a good reference and brings him up-to-date with the latest developments. For the academic surgeon it invites challenges to advance elbow surgery into a new era. The editorial team is proud of what we have been able to produce with the wonderful support of the contributing authors. We thank them for their extremely precious contribution and to ISAKOS for the opportunity to serve the Society in such an important role.

Luigi Pederzini
Greg Bain
Marc Safran

Contents

1 Anatomy and Portals   1
Duncan Thomas McGuire and Gregory Ian Bain

2 Arthroscopic Technique   13
Christian N. Anderson and Marc R. Safran

**3 Osteochondritis Dissecans Lesions and Loose Bodies
of the Elbow**   25
Kevin E. Coates and Gary G. Poehling

4 Arthroscopic Treatment of Lateral Epicondylitis   35
Champ L. Baker Jr and Champ L. Baker III

5 Elbow Arthroscopy in Stiff Elbow   43
Luigi Pederzini, Massimo Tosi, Mauro Prandini and Fabio Nicoletta

6 The Role of Arthroscopy in Elbow Instability   57
Christian N. Anderson and Marc R. Safran

7 Endoscopy Around the Elbow   73
Duncan Thomas McGuire and Gregory Ian Bain

8 Arthroscopic Treatment of Elbow Fractures   83
E. Guerra, A. Marinelli, G. Bettelli, M. Cavaciocchi and R. Rotini

9 Elbow Arthroscopy Complications 103
Graham J. W. King

10 Elbow Arthroscopy: The Future 113
Felix Savoie III and Michael J. O'Brien

Anatomy and Portals

1

Duncan Thomas McGuire and Gregory Ian Bain

1.1 Introduction

Original cadaveric work by Burman in 1932 established that it was possible to introduce an arthroscope into the joint and visualise many aspects of it with relative ease, however it was Andrews and Carson's paper in 1985, Morrey's lectures in 1986 and further Poehling's paper in 1989 that captured the attention of the orthopaedic community [1–4]. A report of 473 cases, demonstrated that all major and cutaneous nerves around the elbow are at risk, with the ulnar nerve most likely to be involved [5]. The risk increased in complex cases, such as in rheumatoid arthritis and capsular releases. A sound working knowledge of the neurovascular anatomy of the elbow and good technique is essential to performing elbow arthroscopy safely.

1.2 Patient Setup

Most surgeons would utilize the *lateral decubitus* position, which was originally described by O'Driscoll and Morrey [6]. The patient is positioned on their side on the table and secured with either a beanbag or bolsters (Fig. 1.1a, b) The arm is placed over a padded bolster, which allows free flexion and extension of the elbow. The anaesthetist has good access to the airway, and the surgeon can mobilize the elbow through its full range, and has access to posterior and anterior compartments

D. T. McGuire · G. I. Bain
Department of Orthopaedics and Trauma, Royal Adelaide Hospital, Adelaide, SA, Australia

G. I. Bain (✉)
Department of Orthopaedics and Trauma, University of Adelaide, Adelaide, SA, Australia
e-mail: greg@gregbain.com.au; gregbain@internode.on.net

L. A. Pederzini (ed.), *Elbow Arthroscopy*,
DOI: 10.1007/978-3-642-38103-4_1, © ISAKOS 2013

Fig. 1.1 a Setup for the
lateral decubitus position.
Note sterile tourniquet. **b** The
site of the patient's tender
lateral epicondyle has been
marked, prior to the
anaesthetic, to ensure that the
correct area is debrided
(Copyright Dr Gregory Bain)

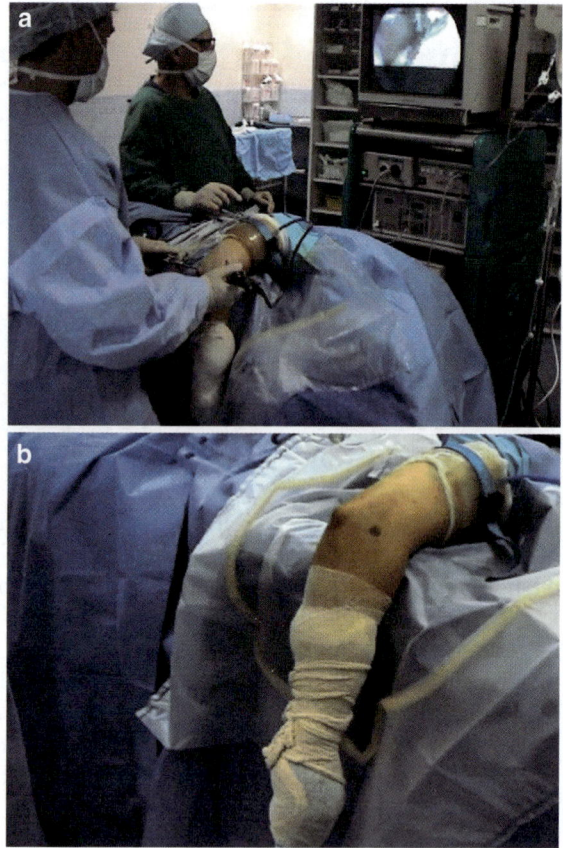

of the joint. However, if an open anterior procedure is required, the patient may
need to be repositioned.

The supine position was first described by Andrews and Carson [2]. The
shoulder is abducted to 90°, the elbow flexed to 90° and the arm suspended by an
overhead traction device. Advantages of this position are that orientation is easier
as the arm is in the anatomical position, the anterior compartment of the elbow is
easily accessed, and the anaesthetist can access the airway. However, access to the
posterior compartment is difficult.

In the *modified supine* position the shoulder is flexed to 90° with the arm across
the chest. This improves access to the posterior compartment when compared to
the standard supine position. There are various mechanical devices available to
suspend the arm across the chest that can be easily adjusted. With the arm across
the chest, the anterior neurovascular structures tend to fall away from the capsule
making work in the anterior compartment easier and safer [7]. The arm may be
removed from the holder and placed on the table if open arthrotomy is required
(Fig. 1.2a, b).

Fig. 1.2 **a** and **b** Setup for
the modified supine position,
the arm is cradled in a gutter
above the patient's chest. The
elbow can be extended and
placed onto a table, to access
to the anterior elbow
(Copyright Dr Gregory Bain)

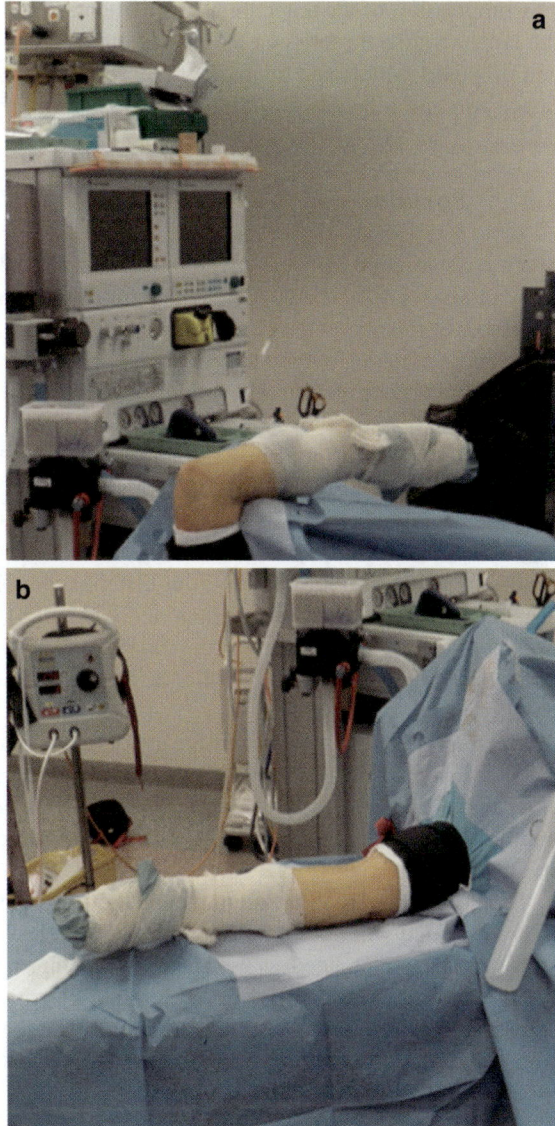

The *prone* position described by Pochling is now not commonly used due to the difficulties of positioning the patient, and due to the fact that the anaesthetist will have difficulty accessing the airway [4].

Elbow arthroscopy can be performed under general anaesthesia or regional block. Some surgeons do not use a regional block so that they can accurately assess the nerve function post-operatively.

Compression of the antecubital fossa is undesirable and thus a 20-degree tilt of the table towards the surgeon may be useful [8]. The bony landmarks, ulnar nerve and proposed portals can be marked before surgery. A tourniquet is placed on the upper arm and inflated just before the surgical procedure is begun.

1.3   Portals

Much consideration has been given to the safe zones for elbow arthroscopy portals and cadaver work has been done to exemplify the neurological relationships about the elbow in relation to the capsule. Care and thought should be given to the site of portal placement to avoid neurovascular injury. Choice of portals depends on surgeon preference and the indication for surgery. Bony landmarks are the guides to making safe entry into the joint.

At the start of the procedure the joint should be distended with normal saline. This may be done via the lateral soft spot of the elbow which is the triangle formed between the lateral epicondyle, the olecranon tip and the radial head. The injection may also be performed posterocentrally into the olecranon fossa with the elbow flexed. Injection of fluid into the joint distends the joint capsule and increases the distance from the bone to the median nerve (12 mm) and radial nerve (6 mm), but does not increase the distance to the ulnar nerve [9, 10]. Injection of fluid into the joint does not change the capsule to nerve distance, which remains in close proximity [9].

Flexion of the elbow increases the average bone to nerve distance, compared to extension, for all nerves: median nerve (5–13 mm), radial nerve (6–10 mm) and ulnar nerve (3–5 mm) [9]. Therefore the elbow should always be flexed and the joint insufflated with fluid to decrease the risk of neurological injury during trochar and cannula insertion (Fig. 1.3a, b).

The normal joint will accommodate 20–30 mL of fluid at 70° of flexion [11]. A contracted joint will have a thicker capsule, have less compliance to distension (by 15 %) and accommodate less fluid (3–9 ml) at approximately 85° [12]. One should avoid over distension of the joint with fluid, which may rupture the joint capsule. Gravity fed fluid inflow is recommended, rather than pressure insufflation via a pump in order to minimize swelling and fluid extravasation into surrounding tissues.

A 30-degree, 4.0 mm arthroscope without a side-venting cannula is preferred to minimize fluid extravasation. A 2.7 mm wrist scope can make visualization of the lateral gutter easier and may be useful in small patients, but is rarely needed. A 70-degree scope may provide benefit in a reduced volume joint [13, 14]. Trocars should be conical and blunt tipped to avoid neurovascular and cartilage injury.

Fig. 1.3 a Cadaver specimen with *pink latex*, which has been injected into the joint. Note the radial nerve lies directly on the anterior capsule over the capitellum and radial head, and that distension increases the distance from the capitellum to the nerve. **b** With elbow flexion, the anterior joint space increases and the neurovascular structures are displaced away from the capitellum. Note however the distance between the radial nerve and the anterior capsule is unchanged with distension and flexion (Copyright Dr Gregory Bain)

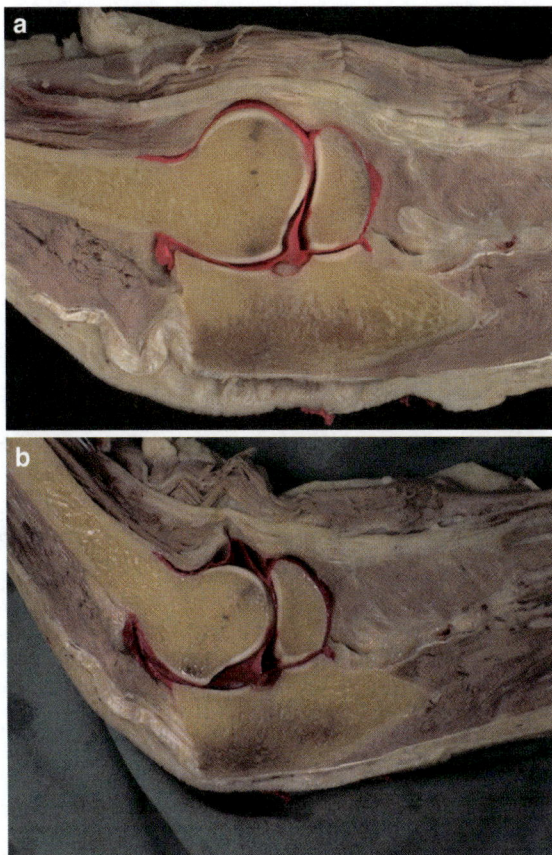

1.3.1 Avoiding Ulnar Nerve Injury

The surgeon should make a habit of identifying the position of the ulnar nerve prior to any skin incision in every patient. The nerve is most at risk with the proximal medial portal, but can be injured with any medial portal, particularly if there has been an ulnar nerve transposition. Normally the nerve is clearly palpable behind the medial epicondyle, so the medial portals can be created knowing the exact position of the nerve. If the nerve is subluxatable, and it can be confidently identified and reduced behind the medial epicondyle, then while it is held reduced the standard technique of proximal medial portal can be used. If the nerve can't be clearly palpated for any reason such as previous ulnar nerve surgery, then a medial incision should be made and the nerve identified before placement of any medial portal [15].

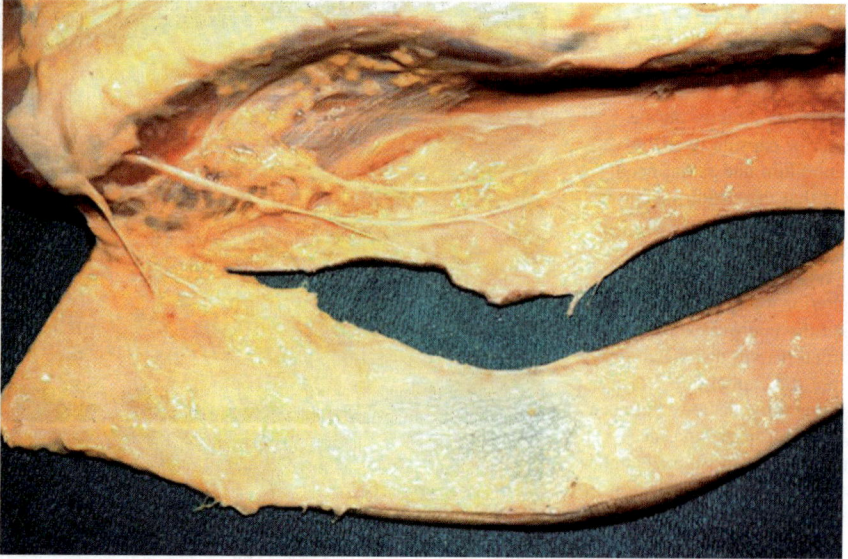

Fig. 1.4 Cadaver dissection demonstrating the cutaneous nerves, which lie in the depths of the subcutaneous fat, on the deep fascia. All of the portals used in elbow arthroscopy, will place the cutaneous nerves at risk. Cutaneous nerve injury can be avoided by a nick in the skin, and then using an artery clip to dissect the subcutaneous fat, before inserting the trochar (Copyright Dr Gregory Bain)

1.3.2 Avoiding Cutaneous Nerve Injury

The authors' preferred method for making portals is the 'nick-and-spread' technique. A 'nick' is made in the skin with a scalpel blade through the dermis, and then a blunt artery forceps is used to dissect the subcutaneous fat to minimize the risk to cutaneous sensory nerves, which are located on the deep fascia in the depths of the subcutaneous tissue [16] (Fig. 1.4). Due to the multiple cutaneous nerves and their branches, there is nearly always a cutaneous nerve within a few millimeters of any portal around the elbow. A trochar is then advanced into the joint. Entry into the joint is confirmed by a backflow of fluid.

Portals may also be created with an 'inside-out' technique using a Wissinger rod. When inserting the trocar for anterior portals the elbow should be flexed to at least 90° to provide maximal clearance of neurovascular structures [17].

1.3.3 Overview of Portal Selection

The authors follow the '2 cm rule'. The working portals are 2 cm proximal to the bony prominences of the elbow.

Anteriorly the working portals are the proximal medial portal and the proximal lateral portal, which are located 2 cm proximal to the medial and lateral epicondyles respectively. Posteriorly the posterocentral and posterolateral portals are located 2 cm proximal to the proximal olecranon.

1.4   Proximal Anteromedial Portal

As described by Poehling [4], the proximal anteromedial portal is a common standard starting portal. This portal provides good visualization of the radial head, coronoid, lateral capsule and gutter. The landmarks for this portal are 2 cm proximal to the medial epicondyle and just anterior to the medial intermuscular septum. The position of the ulnar nerve must be known before creating this portal. The trocar or artery forceps is aimed at the radial head and slid along the anterior aspect of the distal humerus staying on bone deep to the brachialis muscle so as to avoid the median nerve. This portal is used as the starting portal for most surgeons.

At this level the ulnar nerve is 12 mm posterior, the median nerve 12 mm anterior, and the brachial artery 18 mm anterior to the portal [9]. The structure most at risk is the medial antebrachial cutaneous nerve (average of 2.3 mm) [18].

1.5   Proximal Anterolateral Portal

Described by Field et al., this portal is made 1–2 cm proximal to the lateral epicondyle and directly on the anterior humerus [19]. The trocar is aimed towards the centre of the joint and slid along the anterior humerus. It pierces brachioradialis and distal brachialis before entering the joint through the lateral capsule. This portal provides good visualization of the anterior joint and is used by many surgeons as the first portal. The structures at risk are the radial nerve (average 13.7 mm from the portal site) and the posterior branch of the antebrachial cutaneous nerve [average 6.1 mm (range 0–14 mm)] [19]. The proximal anterolateral portal is safer and affords a better visualization of the joint when compared to the other anterolateral portals [20].

1.6   Anteromedial Portal (Accessory Medial Portal)

This portal is made 2 cm distal and 2 cm anterior to the medial epicondyle, which allows excellent visualization of the lateral joint and proximal capsular insertion [8]. The authors use this as the second medial portal and create the portal with a Wissinger rod from lateral to medial. The nerve most at risk is the anterior branch of the medial antebrachial cutaneous nerve (average 1 mm from portal site) [20]. This portal is much safer with the elbow in flexion. The median nerve may lie in direct contact with the cannula with the elbow fully extended. The portal should be created with the elbow in 90° of flexion, as the nerve falls away anteriorly (7–14 mm) [21]. The brachial artery is protected by the thick brachialis muscle (average 15 mm, range 8–20 mm) [20]. This portal should be avoided if there has been an anterior transposition of the ulnar nerve [14]. Although this portal may be hazardous in terms of damage to neurological structures, it offers excellent visualization of the joint.

1.7   Anterolateral Portal

This portal is placed 2 cm distal and 2 cm anterior to the lateral epicondyle. The radial nerve and the posterior antebrachial cutaneous nerve are at risk with the placement of this portal. The trochar is aimed towards the centre of the joint and passes through extensor carpi radialis brevis and supinator muscles. The arthroscope will enter the joint at the sulcus between radial head and capitellum [14]. This portal provides excellent visualization of the lateral and medial aspect of the elbow, with access to the coronoid process, radial head, trochlea and medial capsule. This portal may be placed using an 'outside-in' technique. A needle is inserted through the skin and into the joint. The position of the needle is visualized from within the joint with the arthroscope and the optimal portal position is determined before the skin incision is made. This helps avoid damage to the lateral structures of the joint. Many surgeons prefer to use the proximal anterolateral portal over this portal due to the higher risk of injury to the radial nerve (3 mm) and the posterior antebrachial cutaneous nerve (2 mm) [22]. The arthroscopic cannula may be in contact with both of these nerves during the procedure, particularly if the elbow is in extension [20] (Fig. 1.5).

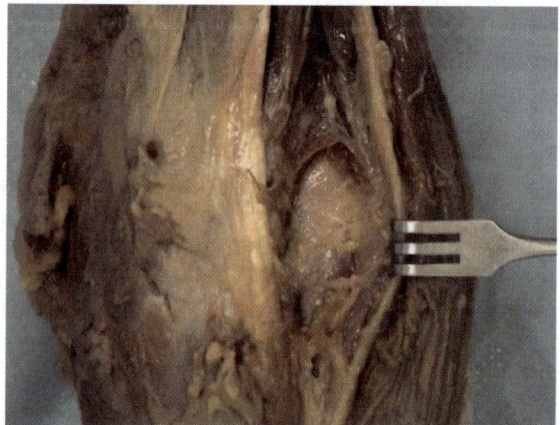

Fig. 1.5 Cadaver dissection of the anterior elbow with the retracted radial nerve lying on the anterior capsule, over the capitellum and radial head (Copyright Dr Gregory Bain)

1.8   Direct Lateral Portal (Soft Spot Portal)

This portal is made in the soft spot on the lateral side of the elbow. The closest neurovascular structure to the portal is the posterior antebrachial cutaneous nerve, (7 mm). This portal allows visualization of the inferior and posterior aspect of the capitellum and the inferior portion of the radioulnar joint.

Multiple lateral portals may be made between the direct lateral portal and the proximal anterolateral portal. These portals allow access to the lateral gutter and may be used to remove loose bodies. These portals are generally safe, however the more distal the portal is made, the higher the risk to the radial nerve. A safe way to make these portals is using the 'outside-in' technique described previously.

1.9   Posterior Portals

Posterior elbow arthroscopy is safer than anterior arthroscopy as the neurovascular structures lie further away. The main two portals used are the posterocentral and the posterolateral portals. These portals allow excellent visualization of the posterior compartment as well as the medial and lateral gutters. These two portals allow retrieval of loose bodies and debridement of osteophytes within the posterior compartment.

The posterocentral portal is made 2 cm proximal to the tip of the olecranon in the midline with the elbow flexed to 90°, by passing through triceps just above its musculotendinous junction. If placed too distal, close to the olecranon tip the triceps tendon may be damaged [17]. The posterior antebrachial cutaneous nerve (23 mm) and the ulnar nerve (25 mm) are unlikely to be injured [14].

The posterolateral portal is made 2 cm proximal to the olecranon tip and at the lateral border of the triceps tendon. For both the posterior portals the trochar is directed towards the olecranon fossa at 45° with the elbow flexed to 90°.

Another posterior portal that has been described is the posterior retractor portal [23]. This portal is made 2 cm proximal to the posterocentral portal and allows insertion of a retractor, which is then used to retract the joint capsule posteriorly and thus aids in visualization of the olecranon fossa.

1.10   Other Instruments

Intra-articular retractors are beneficial and recommended by several authors [13, 23]. Their use aids visualization in the joint by retracting the anterior capsule and synovium, and hence decreases the need to use higher pressure insufflation for improving visualization, which decreases swelling around the joint (Fig. 1.6).

Burrs and resectors are often required, but care should be taken to only employ them under direct vision. The resectors should be directed away from neurological structures when they are in use. Free drainage rather than suction should be used,

Fig. 1.6 The back end of mini Hoffman retractors may be used as intra-articular retractors which aids visualization inside the joint. They may be used together, passed from side to side (Copyright Dr Gregory Bain)

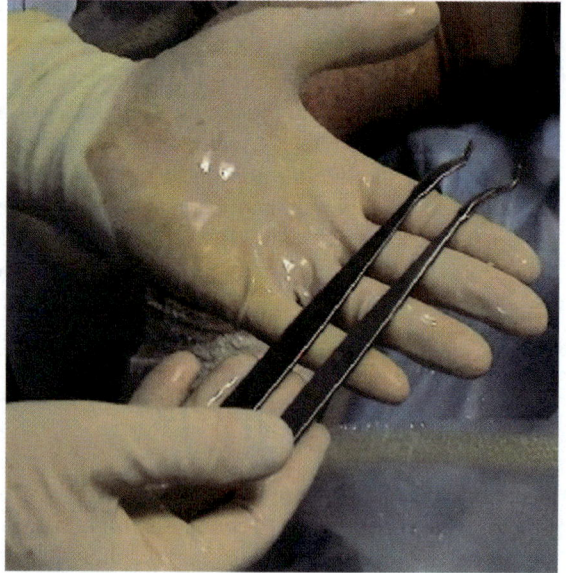

and the resectors should have no teeth to avoid catching soft tissue in the aperture of the resector. This will minimize the chance of inadvertent damage to nerves during débridement or capsulectomy.

References

1. Burman S (1932) Arthroscopy of the elbow joint: a cadaver study. J Bone Joint Surg Am 14:349–350
2. Andrews JR, Carson WG (1985) Arthroscopy of the elbow. Arthroscopy 1(2):97–107
3. Morrey BF (1986) Arthrosocpy of the elbow. Instr Course Lect 35:102–107
4. Poehling GG, Whipple TL, Sisco L, Goldman B (1989) Elbow arthroscopy: a new technique. Arthroscopy 5(3):222–224
5. Kelly EW, Morrey BF, O'Driscoll SW (2001) Complications of elbow arthroscopy. J Bone Joint Surg Am 83(1):25–34
6. O'Driscoll SW, Morrey BF (1992) Arthroscopy of the elbow: diagnostic and therapeutic benefits and hazards. J Bone Joint Surg Am 74(1):84–94
7. Dodson CC, Nho SJ, Williams RJ 3rd, Altchek DW (2008) Elbow arthroscopy. J Am Acad Orthop Surg 16(10):574–585
8. Steinmann S (2007) Elbow arthroscopy: where are we now? Arthroscopy 23(11):1231–1236
9. Miller CD, Jobe CM, Wright MH (1995) Neuroanatomy in elbow arthroscopy. J Shoulder Elbow Surg 4(3):168–174
10. Miller D, Gregory JJ, Hay SM (2008) Arthroscopy of the elbow. Current Orthop. 22:104–110
11. O'Driscoll SW, Morrey BF, An KN (1990) Intraarticular pressure and capacity of the elbow. Arthroscopy 6(2):100–103
12. Gallay SH, Richards RR, O'Driscoll SW (1993) Intraarticular capacity and compliance of stiff and normal elbows. Arthroscopy 9(1):9–13

13. Watts AC, Bain GI (2010) New techniques in elbow arthroscopy. In: Savoie FH, Field LD (eds) AANA advanced arthroscopy: the elbow and wrist. Saunders-Elsevier, Philadelphia, pp 124–131

14. Abboud JA, Ricchetti ET, Tjoumakaris F, Ramsey ML (2006) Elbow arthroscopy: basic setup and portal placement. J Am Acad Orthop Surg 14(5):312–318

15. Sahajpal DT, Bionna D, O'Driscoll SW (2010) Anteromedial elbow arthroscopy portals in patients with prior ulnar nerve transposition or subluxation. Arthroscopy 26(8):1045–1052

16. Dowdy PA, Bain GI, King GJ, Patterson SD (1995) The midline posterior elbow incision. An anatomical appraisal. J Bone Joint Surg Br 77(5):696–699

17. Moskal MJ, Savoie FH 3rd, Field LD (1999) Elbow arthroscopy in trauma and reconstruction. Orthop Clin North Am 30(1):163–177

18. O'Holleran JD, Altchek DW (2006) Elbow arthroscopy: treatment of the thrower's elbow. Instr Course Lect 55:95–107

19. Field LD, Altchek DW, Warren RF, O'Brien SJ, Skyhar MJ, Wickiewicz TL (1994) Arthroscopic anatomy of the lateral elbow: a comparison of three portals. Arthroscopy 10(6):602–607

20. Stothers K, Day B, Regan WR (1995) Arthroscopy of the elbow: anatomy, portal sites, and a description of the proximal lateral portal. Arthroscopy 11(4):449–457

21. Unlu MC, Kesmezacar H, Akgun I, Ogut T, Uzun I (2006) Anatomic relationship between elbow arthroscopy portals and neurovascular structures in different elbow and forearm positions. J Shoulder Elbow Surg 15(4):457–462

22. Lynch GJ, Meyers JF, Whipple TL, Caspari RB (1986) Neurovascular anatomy and elbow arthroscopy: inherent risks. Arthroscopy 2(3):190–197

23. Steinmann SP, King GJ, Savoie FH 3rd (2006) Arthroscopic treatment of the arthritic elbow. Instr Course Lect 55:109–117

Arthroscopic Technique

2

Christian N. Anderson and Marc R. Safran

2.1 Anesthesia

Regional or general anesthesia can be used for arthroscopy of the elbow and each has advantages and disadvantages. Regional anesthesia most commonly involves the use of a brachial plexus block, which has the advantage of providing excellent post-operative pain control while minimizing use of narcotics. Regional anesthesia is also preferred for patients with co-morbidities that preclude the use of general anesthesia. The most significant disadvantage of using a regional block is that it prevents accurate neurologic assessment of the extremity post-operatively. Patients may also become apprehensive or uncomfortable during surgery, either from the procedure or the positioning required for surgery, and conversion to general anesthesia may become necessary. The overall complication rate for interscalene brachial plexus blocks has been estimated at 1.1 % [3]. Although relatively rare, serious and disabling complications include central nervous system, respiratory, and cardiovascular compromise, as well as permanent nerve deficit [3]. A Bier Block may also be used for regional anesthesia during elbow arthroscopy, but is less desirable because tourniquet pressure can cause significant patient discomfort and there is a small risk of systemic toxicity if the tourniquet is suddenly deflated after introduction of the intravenous anesthetic.

Many surgeons prefer general anesthesia because it allows improved patient comfort and total muscle relaxation, which prevents patient movement during surgery, and avoids complications associated with a regional block. The disadvantages of general anesthesia include longer post-operative recovery and potentially greater pain in the immediate post-operative period.

C. N. Anderson · M. R. Safran (✉)
Stanford University, 450 Broadway Street, M/C 6342, Redwood City,
CA 94063, USA
e-mail: msafran@stanford.edu; lockshin@stanford.edu

L. A. Pederzini (ed.), *Elbow Arthroscopy*,
DOI: 10.1007/978-3-642-38103-4_2, © ISAKOS 2013

2.2   Positioning

For arthroscopic elbow surgery, the patient may be positioned supine, lateral decubitus, or prone depending on surgeon preference and location of the pathology. Several important principles should be followed during positioning. All bony prominences should be well padded, and the surgeon should have circumferential access to the elbow region. Positioning should allow unimpeded elbow flexion for safe portal placement, complete evaluation of intra-articular anatomy, and maximal distension of the joint capsule [7]. The use of a sterile tourniquet allows greater access to the elbow and provides excellent visualization, allowing a safe and efficient procedure.

2.2.1   Supine

The supine position was originally described by Andrews and Carson in 1985 [2]. The patient is placed supine with the shoulder at the lateral edge of the operating table in 90° of abduction, and the elbow flexed to 90°. The forearm is secured in a prefabricated wrist gauntlet or finger traps, and traction is applied with a pulley system to allow joint distraction (Fig. 2.1). Positioning a patient supine has several advantages. Firstly, the elbow is maintained in the normal anatomic position relative to the surgeon, allowing improved orientation. Secondly, it allows a relatively quick set up and provides the anesthesiologist with direct access to the patient's airway. Additionally, if an open procedure is indicated, traction can be easily released and the arm can be placed on an arm board. The disadvantages are that arthroscopically accessing the posterior compartment of the elbow from this position is difficult and anatomic orientation posteriorly can be more challenging. Additionally, the traction set up may risk the sterility of the field, add cost to the procedure, and may not provide enough stability to the arm during instrumentation, necessitating an additional assistant to hold the arm.

2.2.2   Lateral Decubitus

The lateral decubitus position was first utilized by O'Driscoll and Morrey [6] because it offers increased stability and access to the arm and unrestricted elbow motion, compared to the supine position. The lateral decubitus position also allows easy access to the patient's airway by the anesthesiologist. In this position, the patient is placed on the operating table with the operative extremity upward and the torso/pelvis stabilized with a beanbag or hip positioners. An axillary role is then placed, and the patient is secured to the table with straps or tape. The operative arm is supported by an appropriately padded bolster, with the shoulder flexed and internally rotated 90° and the elbow in 90° of flexion (Fig. 2.2). The bolster should be placed proximal to the antecubital fossa and high enough to

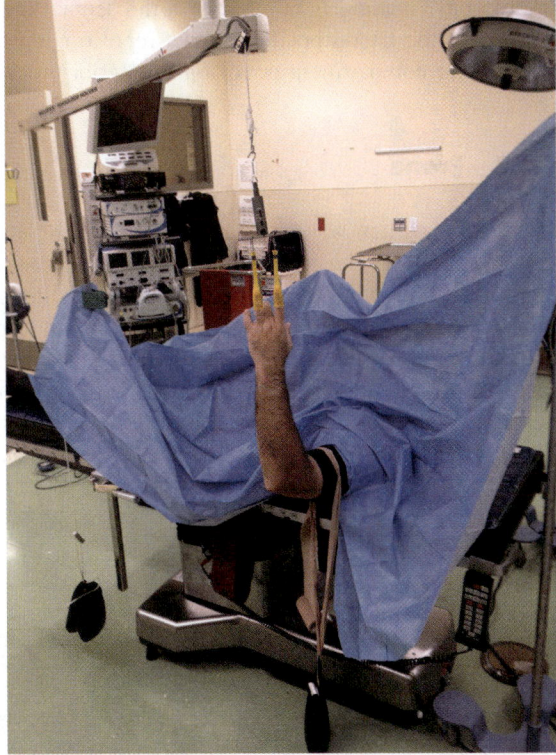

Fig. 2.1 The supine position. The arm is held upright with finger traps and a traction system. A counter weight can be added to the arm to provide additional joint distraction

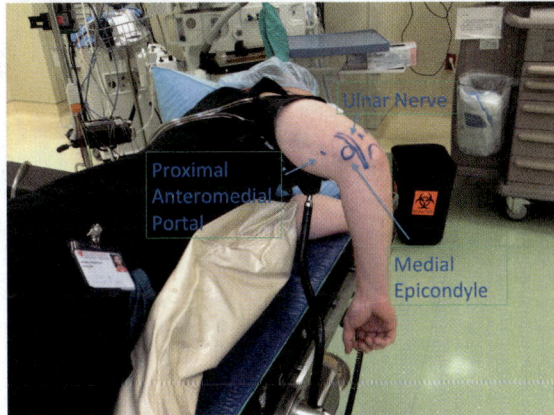

Fig. 2.2 The lateral decubitus position. The patient is held in this position with a beanbag and the operative extremity is rested over a padded bolster

prevent compression of the anterior neurovascular structures, allow maximal distention of the joint capsule, and allow unrestricted elbow motion. The contra-lateral shoulder and elbow should be placed on an arm board with enough flexion to not interfere with elbow flexion of the operative extremity. This position of the elbow, with the olecranon up, is similar to the position of the knee for knee arthroscopy, making it familiar to arthroscopic knee surgeons. The main disadvantage of the lateral position is that repositioning may be required for access to the anterior compartment or for open anterior procedures.

2.2.3 Prone

The prone position was popularized by Poehling et al. [8] in 1989. After undergoing general anesthesia, the patient is placed prone near the edge of the table on chest rolls. The shoulder is abducted to 90° and the upper arm is supported with an arm board or holder, allowing elbow flexion and gravity distraction of the joint (Fig. 2.3a and b). The elbow should undergo a full range of motion to make sure there are no blocks to flexion or extension. The prone position offers the similar advantages and disadvantages compared to the lateral decubitus position; however, patient positioning can be more cumbersome, and access to the airway is limited.

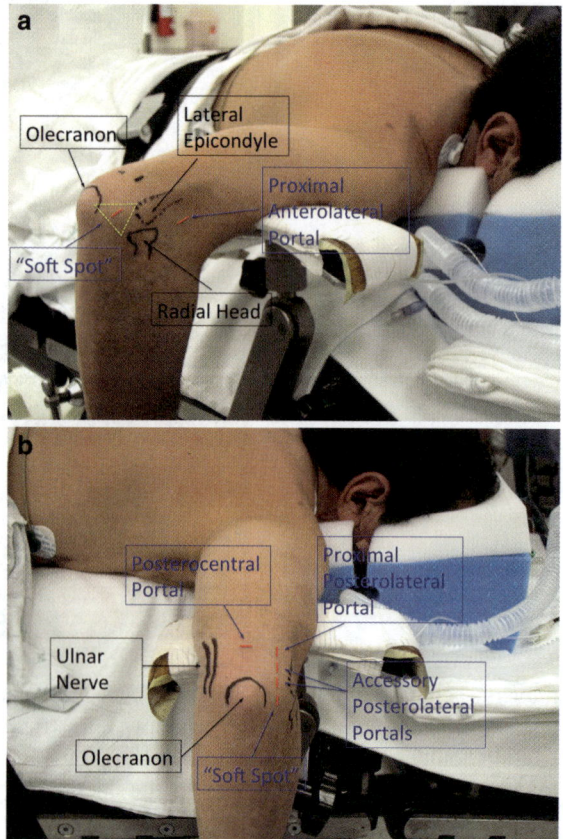

Fig. 2.3 The prone position. The patient is placed on chest rolls and the operative extremity is rested over a padded bolster.
a Demonstrates the "soft spot" and proximal anterolateral portals.
b Demonstrates the posterocentral, proximal posterolateral, accessory posterolateral, and "soft spot" portals

2.3   Set-Up and Instrumentation

The general set-up places the arthroscopic tower, pump, and mechanical shaver system on the opposite side of the table from the surgeon and operative extremity (Fig. 2.4). After positioning the patient, the skin of the operative extremity is prepared with a chlorahexidine disinfectant solution and draped with enough room to allow placement of the sterile tourniquet (Fig. 2.5). An elastic wrap is placed

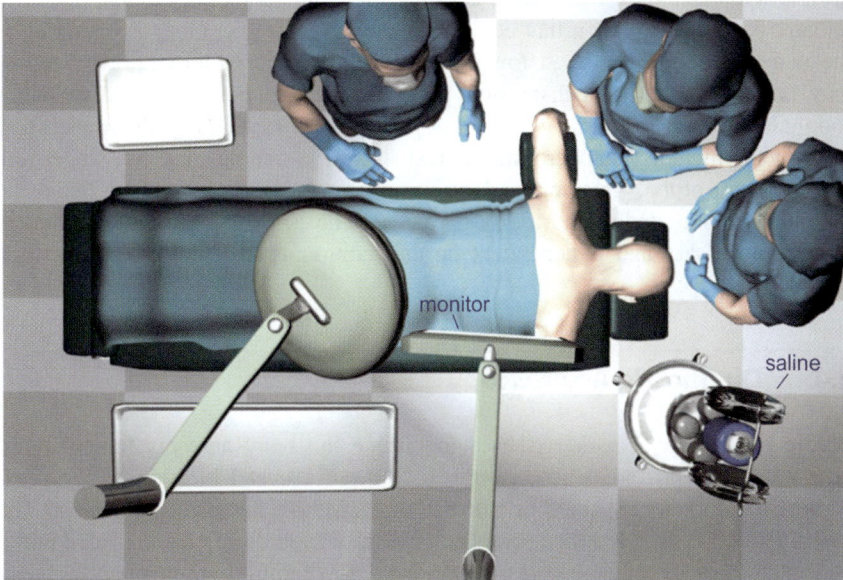

Fig. 2.4 General room set-up

Fig. 2.5 The operative extremity is prepped and draped high enough to allow a sterile tourniquet to be placed without interfering with portal placement and instrumentation

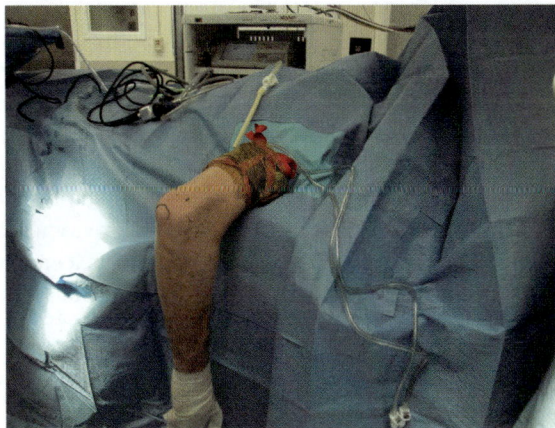

circumferentially around the hand and forearm to minimize fluid extravasation into the soft tissues.

Standard equipment necessary for shoulder and knee arthroscopy can be utilized for elbow arthroscopy. A 4 mm arthroscope with a 30° lens is most commonly used and allows a wide field of view and adequate fluid flow. A 4 mm 70° and 2.7 mm arthroscope should be available if viewing becomes difficult through the standard equipment or for smaller patients. An interchangeable cannula system can be used to minimize tissue damage and fluid extravasation when changing the viewing portal or switching arthroscopes. Because of the close proximity of the intra-articular pathology and joint capsule, the cannula should be non-vented to prevent fluid extravasation that could occur when the camera lens is operating at the margin of the capsule. A low-pressure arthroscopic pump or gravity inflow may be used to for joint distension. If an mechanical pump is used, pressures should be kept at <30 mm Hg to prevent joint capsule rupture [7]. Other necessary instruments include a standard mechanical shaver, switching stick, Wissinger rod, blunt trocar, probe, grasping and biting instruments, straight blunt hemostat, 18 gauge spinal needle, and a 30 cc syringe. The use of specialized equipment may be necessary and is dependent on the requirements of the procedure to be performed.

2.4   Diagnostic Arthroscopy

Before beginning, a marker is used to outline the bony anatomy (epicondyles, olecranon tip, and radial head), arthroscopic portals, and location of the ulnar nerve. The ulnar nerve should be palpated during elbow flexion and extension, and if subluxation is detected the nerve should be protected during medial sided portal placement. For surgeons with less experience, it is helpful to remember the radial head is always on the cephalad side of the elbow for orientation purposes.

After inflation of the tourniquet to 250 mm Hg, the joint is then injected with 25 ml of physiologic saline to allow full distension of the capsule [7] and shift the neurovascular structures away from the joint [5]. This puncture is administered through the "soft spot" located between the tip of the olecranon, radial head, and lateral epicondyle (Fig. 2.3a and b). Intra-articular placement of the saline is confirmed by slight extension and supination of the arm that occurs with capsular inflation. Removing the syringe from the needle will demonstrate fluid backflow from the needle, also confirming intra-articular fluid placement. After introduction of fluid into the joint, arthroscopic portals can be placed in a systematic manner. Flexing the elbow relaxes the anterior neurovascular structures and places them at less risk of damage during anterior portal placement [5]. All incisions should be through the skin only to avoid damage to cutaneous nerves, followed by a blunt straight hemostat or trocar for joint penetration.

The elbow can be viewed as having three separate compartments: anterior, posterior, and posterolateral, and during a diagnostic arthroscopy each compartment should undergo evaluation. There is still controversy regarding which portal to create first and is dependent on surgeon preference, location of pathology, and location of portals relative to neurovascular structures. The senior author prefers to start with the proximal anteromedial portal, followed by the proximal anterolateral portal. After the anterior compartment arthroscopy using the two aforementioned portals, posterior compartment arthroscopy is performed using proximal posterolateral and posterocentral portals made at the same time. When necessary, the direct lateral (soft spot) portal is then made.

2.4.1 Anterior Compartment

We begin the diagnostic arthroscopy in the anterior compartment with the *proximal anteromedial portal* because cadaveric studies have shown it to be further from major neurovascular structures relative to other starting portals [4, 11]. The starting point for this portal is located 2 cm proximal to the medial humeral epicondyle and anterior to the intermuscular septum, which usually can be palpated (Fig. 2.2) [8]. After making the skin incision, a blunt trocar inside an arthroscopic cannula is used to palpate and stay anterior on the shaft of the distal humerus. The trocar is directed to the center of the ventral surface of the joint and driven trough the capsule. Intra-articular placement is confirmed with fluid backflow upon removal of the trocar from the sheath. If the patient has a history of ulnar nerve transposition or medial sided elbow surgery, identification of the location of the nerve should be determined before placing the cannula. If the location of the nerve cannot be established, a 2–3 cm skin incision should be used to dissect directly down to the capsule, allowing safe portal placement [10].

After the portal is placed and the trochar is removed from the cannula, the arthroscope is introduced and the anterior compartment is systematically examined. The radial head serves as an important landmark and the articular surface should be evaluated with pronation-supination of the forearm. The annular ligament is evaluated along the radial neck. The arthroscope is next directed anterosuperiorly to evaluate the capitellum and radial fossa (Fig. 2.6a). Advancing the scope from here allows inspection of the lateral gutter, lateral capsule, and origin of extensor muscles to the lateral epicondyle. The anterior portions of the capsule are examined as the camera is withdrawn medially. The arthroscope is then used to inspect the proximal radio-ulnar joint, coronoid process, coronoid fossa, and trochlea (Fig. 2.6b).

After evaluation of the anterior compartment, a *proximal anterolateral portal* is established 2 cm proximal and 1 cm anterior to the lateral epicondyle (Fig. 2.3a) [11]. This portal is made using an "outside in" technique by directing an 18 gauge needle towards the central portion of the joint. Once the appropriate placement and trajectory of the needle is established, the skin only is incised and either a blunt

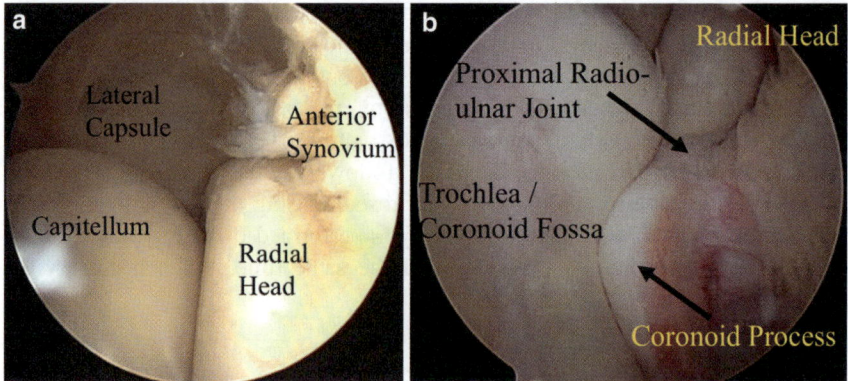

Fig. 2.6 Arthroscopic anatomy of the anterolateral (**a**) and anterior (**b**) elbow viewed from the proximal anteromedial portal

straight hemostat or blunt trocar/arthroscopic cannula is advanced through the brachioradialis into the anterior compartment of the elbow. This portal can be used for instrumentation when viewing from the proximal anteromedial portal and for viewing the ventral and medial aspect of the joint. Anatomic structures that can be viewed are similar to what can be seen through medial portals; however, the proximal anterolateral portal allows improved visualization of the medial capsule and anterior bundle of the medial collateral ligament but a lesser view of the radiocapitellar and medial ulnohumeral joints [1]. Of note, the anterolateral portal is close to the radial nerve, particularly the posterior interosseous nerve. The more proximal the lateral portal is, the greater the distance from the radial nerve, increasing the margin of safety.

Procedures that can be performed in the anterior compartment of the elbow from the proximal anteromedial and anterolateral portals include diagnosis of ulnar collateral ligament insufficiency, removal of ventral loose bodies and osteophytes, synovectomy for rheumatoid arthritis or synovial proliferative disorders, debridement and microfracture of osteochondral lesions, capsular release for arthrofibrosis, arthroscopically assisted internal fixation of radial head fractures, radial head excision, and debridement of the extensor carpi radialis brevis tendon for lateral epicondylitis. Ventral loose bodies often "hide" at the proximal radioulnar joint.

2.4.2 Posterior Compartments

Following completion of anterior joint arthroscopy, we routinely perform posterior compartment arthroscopy. A *posterocentral "trans-tricipital" portal* is useful for evaluating the proximal portions of posterior compartment. To make this portal a horizontal skin incision is made in-line with Langer's lines 3 cm above the tip of the olecranon (Fig. 2.3b). Once the skin has been incised, the blade is turned 90° and the triceps tendon is punctured in-line with its fibers. The elbow is placed in 30–45° of flexion and a blunt trocar/cannula is advanced toward the olecranon fossa until the joint capsule is penetrated. Next, the *proximal posterolateral portal* is made lateral to the trans-tricipital portal on the lateral border of the triceps tendon (Fig. 2.3b) [2]. After making the skin incision, a blunt trochar and sheath are introduced into the olecranon fossa. If visualization is obscured after first entering the olecranon fossa, a mechanical shaver can be used through the trans-tricipital portal to debride any soft tissues occupying the field of view. This is safe if the instruments are in the olecranon fossa.

Both of these portals allow visualization of the posterior trochlea, tip of the olecranon, olecranon fossa, and the lateral and medial gutters/capsule (Fig. 2.7a, b, and c). The ulnar nerve is located superficial to the joint capsule and posterior bundle of the ulnar collateral ligament in the medial gutter; therefore, caution should be used when debriding this area to prevent nerve injury [8].

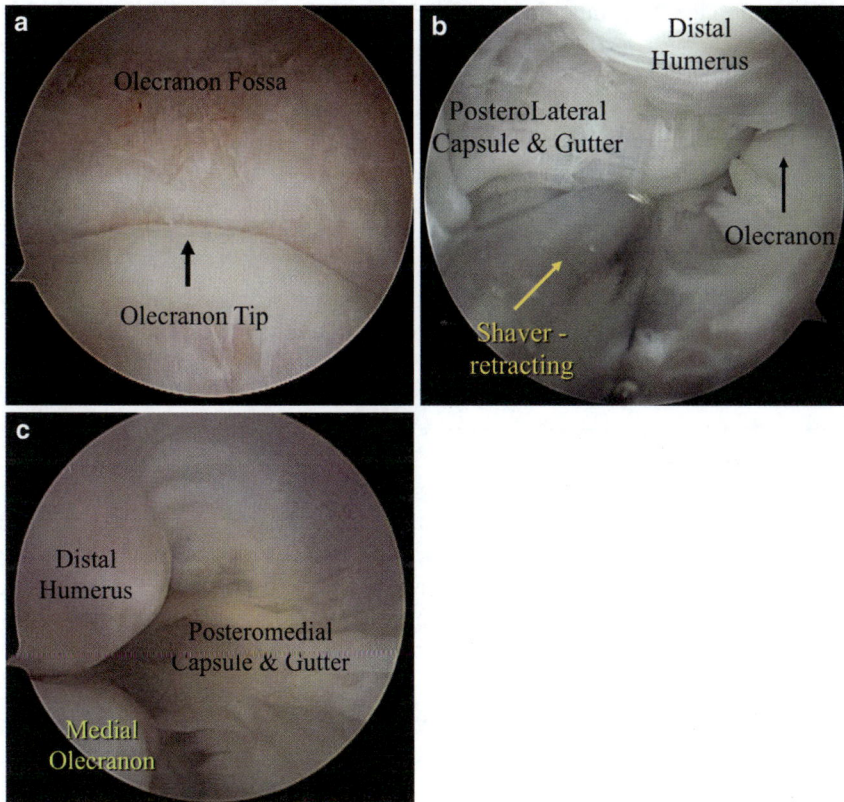

Fig. 2.7 Arthroscopic anatomy of the posterior elbow viewed from the posterocentral portal. Viewing centrally (**a**), laterally (**b**), and medially (**c**) with the 30° arthroscope

The proximal posterolateral and trans-tricipital portals can be used together as viewing and instrumentation portals for treating a variety of conditions including removal of loose bodies and osteophytes, posterior joint synovectomy, joint arthrolysis, and debridement of osteochondral and osteochondritis dissecans (OCD) lesions.

In cases of posterolateral plica or OCD of the capitellum, a *direct lateral* (*soft spot*) *portal* that was used to insufflate the joint can be made for visualization (Fig. 2.3a and b). From this portal, the posterior portions of the radiocapitellar joint, radial head, and dorsal capitellum are inspected. Again, the forearm can be pronated and supinated for identification of the radial head. The camera lens is then directed medially to evaluate the posterior radioulnar joint, followed by the ulnohumeral articulation and tip of the olecranon. A blunt trochar or Wissinger rod may be introduced from either of the posterior portals and placed between the ulna and distal humerus to open this articulation for visualization [9]. *Accessory posterolateral portals* can be created superiorly inline with the direct lateral portal to allow instrumentation for the treatment of OCD lesions of the capitellum and removal of loose bodies (Fig. 2.3b). When treating pathology in the posterolateral space one can also switch to the 2.7 mm arthroscope to prevent instrument crowding.

Through the aforementioned anterior and posterior portals combined, 90 % of the radiocapitellar joint and 75 % of the humeral articular surface is visible [1]. Without the joint jack maneuver, 25 % of the ulnar articular surface can be seen, but with the opening of the joint with the blunt instrument, more than half of the ulnohumeral articular surface can be visualized.

Following the completion of the arthroscopic procedure, some surgeons inject anesthetic into the elbow for postoperative pain relief; however, others prefer not to inject anesthetic to allow for neurovascular examination in the recovery room. After completion of the procedure, the elbow is usually dressed with a temporary bulky dressing for 2–4 days, followed by early active range of motion exercises, unless immobilization is required.

2.5 Summary

Although technically demanding, elbow arthroscopy has emerged as an effective method to diagnose and treat a wide variety of pathologic conditions about the elbow. Knowledge of arthroscopic anatomy and a systematic approach to set-up, positioning, portal placement, and diagnostic arthroscopy are important to a successful intervention and in avoiding complications.

References

1. Adolfsson L (1994) Arthroscopy of the elbow joint: a cadaveric study of portal placement. J Shoulder Elbow Surg 3:53–61
2. Andrews JR, Carson WG (1985) Arthroscopy of the elbow. Arthroscopy 1:97–107

3. Lenters TR, Davies J, Matsen III FA (2007) The types and severity of complications associated with interscalene brachial plexus block anesthesia: local and national evidence. J Shoulder Elbow Surg 16:379–387
4. Lindenfeld TN (1990) Medial approach in elbow arthroscopy. Am J Sports Med 18:413–417
5. Lynch GJ, Meyers JF, Whipple TL, Caspari RB (1986) Neurovascular anatomy and elbow arthroscopy: inherent risks. Arthroscopy 2:190–197
6. O'Driscoll SW, Morrey BF (1992) Arthroscopy of the elbow. Diagnostic and therapeutic benefits and hazards. J Bone Joint Surg (Am) 74:84–94
7. O'Driscoll SW, Morrey BF, An KN (1990) Intraarticular pressure and capacity of the elbow. Arthroscopy 6:100–103
8. Poehling GG, Whipple TL, Sisco L, Goldman B (1989) Elbow arthroscopy: a new technique. Arthroscopy 5:222–224
9. Selby RM, O'brien SJ, Kelly AM, Drakos M (2002) The joint jack. Arthroscopy 18:440–445
10. Steinmann SP (2007) Elbow arthroscopy: where are we now? Arthroscopy 23:1231–1236
11. Stothers K, Day B, Regan WR (1995) Arthroscopy of the elbow: anatomy, portal sites, and a description of the proximal lateral portal. Arthroscopy 11:449–457

Osteochondritis Dissecans Lesions and Loose Bodies of the Elbow

3

Kevin E. Coates and Gary G. Poehling

3.1 Introduction

Ostochondritis dissecans (OCD) lesions consist of a localized portion of the articular surface separating from the underlying bone [1]. Elbow OCD lesions typically occur in the capitellum of the dominant upper extremity. These injuries typically occur in adolescent baseball players and gymnasts, likely due to the repetitive overhead activity and upper extremity weight bearing performed in these sports [2–5].

The most common location of an elbow OCD is the capitellum, located centrally or anterolaterally. The pathomechanics of the lesion is thought to be repetitive microtrauma to the subchondral bone leading to microfracture and compromised circulation. The decrease in circulation then leads to separation of the cartilage from the subchondral bone and formation of loose bodies. The humeral capitellum has a tenuous blood flow resulting from a low number of feeding capillaries, perhaps leading to this being the most frequent location of OCD lesions in the elbow [1].

3.2 Diagnosis

The typical presentation of a patient with a capitellar OCD is child between the ages of 10 and 15 years old. The patient typically presents with an insidious onset of pain. The chief complaints are usually pain, tenderness and swelling over the lateral aspect of the elbow. The most frequently encountered patient is a male

K. E. Coates (✉) · G. G. Poehling
Department of Orthopaedic Surgery, Wake Forest Baptist Medical Center,
Winston-Salem, NC, USA
e-mail: kcoates@wakehealth.edu

G. G. Poehling
e-mail: poehling@wakehealth.edu

L. A. Pederzini (ed.), *Elbow Arthroscopy*,
DOI: 10.1007/978-3-642-38103-4_3, © ISAKOS 2013

baseball pitcher with the symptoms present in the dominant upper extremity. Gymnasts also represent a high percentage of capitellar OCD patients. The patient may present with loss of terminal extension and with mechanical symptoms if late in the disease process [5].

Physical exam findings may include loss of motion, tendnerness and a positive radiocapitellar compression test. This test is performed by placing the elbow into full extension and providing an axial load while performing pronation and supination of the forearm. If the test results in mechanical symptoms, it is considered positive for an OCD [6].

One must differentiate between osteochondritis dissecans and osteochondrosis of the capitellum (Panner's Disesase), as they often present with similar symptoms. Patients that have osteochondrosis present between the ages of 7–12 and have a self limited course. Observation and rest is the treatment of choice for osteochondrosis, and most patients have a complete resolution with recalcification of the capitellum on radiographs within one year [7–9].

As the natural progression of an OCD lesion is to produce a loose fragment, one needs to differentiate between a stable and unstable fragment. Perhaps more importantly, stable lesions may heal with non-operative management, while unstable lesions require surgical management to address [2]. Patient factors suggesting a stable lesion include skeletal immaturity, nearly normal range of motion, and flattening of subchondral bone [3, 9–11].

3.3   Imaging

The first line in diagnostic imaging is plain radiograph evaluation. Unfortunately, plain radiographs may be normal, or show only minimal changes in the early stages of the process. Figure 3.1 represents the lateral projection of a patient with a capitellar OCD. The localized findings can be used to distinguish an OCD lesion from the global effects of osteochondrosis on the capitellum as shown in Fig. 3.2. Figure 3.3 shows the same osteochondrosis lesion at 1-year follow up, demonstrating the complete resolution of the lesion with normal calcification of the capitellum.

A computed tomography (CT) scan may be used to evaluate for presence of loose bodies. Both standard two-dimensional and three-dimensional CT scans can be used to show presence of loose bodies.

The imaging modality of choice for early detection of OCD lesions with normal plain radiographs, however, is MRI. The use of MRI allows evaluation of the chondral surface and can help differentiate between stable and unstable lesions. Two recent studies have reported high sensitivity for MRI in detecting unstable lesions. The reported sensitivities ranged from 84 to 100 % using the staging criteria of De Smet et al., Dipaola et al. and Kijowski et al. However, the specificity was found to be quite low using the criteria by De Smet et al. and Dipaola et al. reaching only 44 % [12–15].

Fig. 3.1 Lateral radiograph showing a capitellar OCD lesion. *Note* the irregular surface at the tip of the *white arrow*. Just anterior to the arrow is the loose body

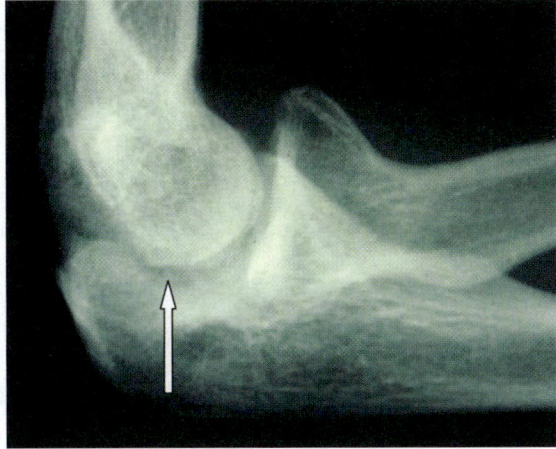

Fig. 3.2 AP radiograph showing osteochondrosis of the capitellum

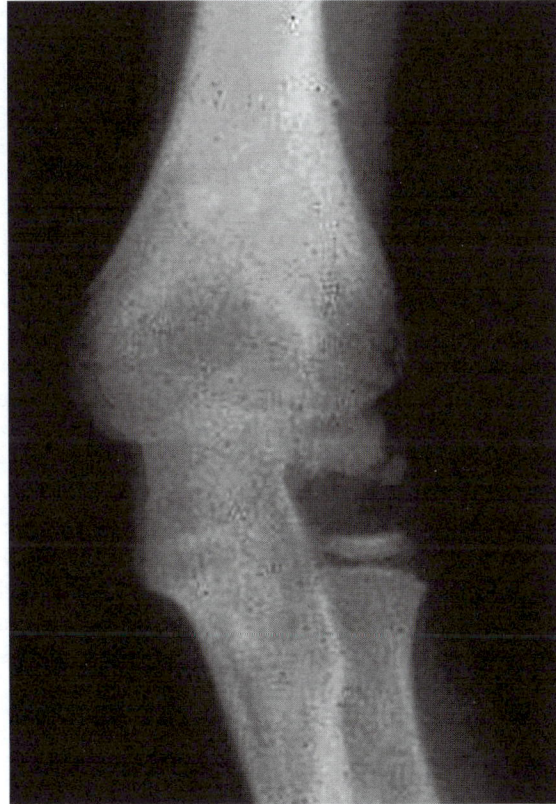

Fig. 3.3 AP radiograph of
the same elbow as Fig. 3.2
one year later showing
complete resolution

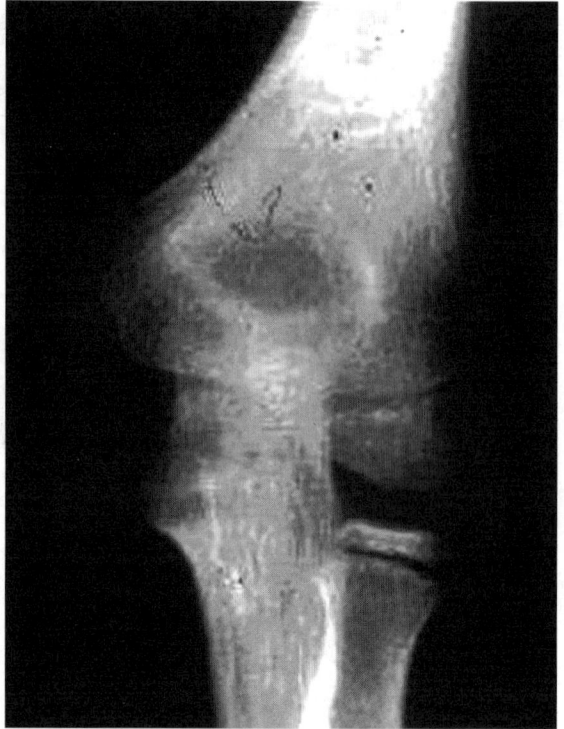

3.4   Management

Treatment for stable, early stage OCD lesions is cessation of repetitive stress on
the elbow and observation. If the lesion has not resolved in 3–6 months, then
consideration of surgical management is made [2].

Surgical management is the treatment of choice for unstable lesions, lesions
that have failed non-operative management and loose bodies. Lesions that are
unstable have a tendency to remain symptomatic even if no loose body is present,
therefore lending to the recommendation for surgery.

A recently published study presents another criteria to consider when deciding
between operative versus non-operative management. The study by Shi et al.
proposed classifying lesions as not only stable versus unstable, but also contained
versus uncontained. They found that uncontained lesions had greater flexion
contractures preoperatively and postoperatively and were associated with higher
rates of joint effusions [16].

3.5 Surgery

Arthroscopic management of OCD lesions has been shown to provide excellent results with high patient satisfaction and no progressive loss of motion [9]. It is our recommendation to proceed with arthroscopic management as a first line treatment with open procedures as a secondary option for failure of arthroscopy.

The patient is placed in the lateral position using a bean-bag positioner. The operative limb is held in place using a modified arm holder as shown in Fig. 3.4. No tourniquet is used for the procedure and an arthroscopic pump with pressure monitoring is used for infusion. The mainstay working portals are the proximal medial and the anterior lateral portals. Motorized shavers and loose body grasping forceps are also used.

The proximal medial portal is created first and the arthroscope introduced into the joint. This portal is placed 2 cm proximal to the medial epicondyle and just anterior to the medial intermuscular septum, thus protecting the ulnar nerve. It is important to maintain contact with the anterior humerus while placing the sheath to avoid injuring the median nerve and brachial artery [17]. The anatomy of the proximal medial portal can be seen in Fig. 3.5.

Using an inside out technique, the anterior lateral portal is then created. With the arthroscope remaining in the proximal medial portal, a diagnostic arthroscopy of the anterior joint is then performed. If anterior pathology is identified, the instruments are passed through the anterior lateral portal to perform debridement and removal of any loose bodies encountered.

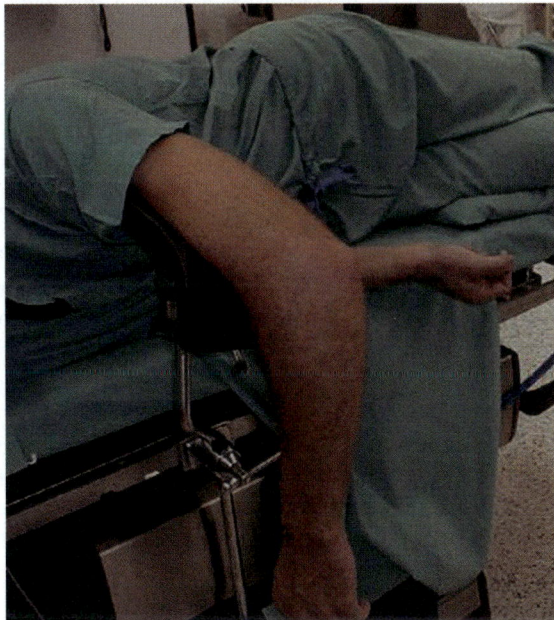

Fig. 3.4 Patient positioning for elbow arthroscopy

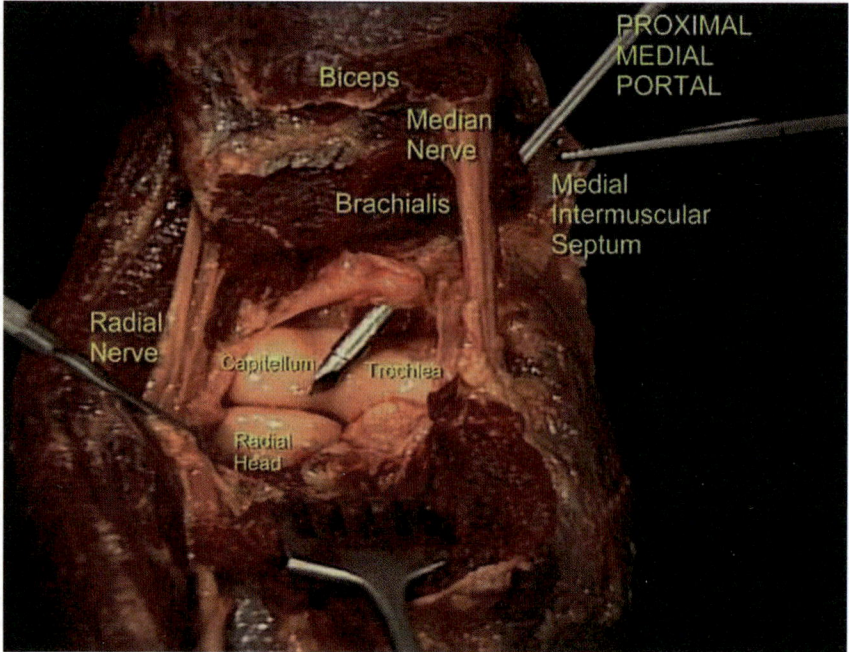

Fig. 3.5 Anatomy of the proximal medial portal as described by Poehling et al. [17]. Please note that the brachialis protects both the median and radial nerves

To assist in management of lesions, a mid lateral or adjacent portal may be used. The mid lateral portal is located at the center of a triangle made by the lateral epicondyle, radial head and tip of the olecranon. The adjacent portal is dependent on the lesion to be addressed and is localized with a needle anywhere in the posterior lateral elbow.

Once any anterior lesions are addressed, the arthroscope is redirected into the posterolateral portal. From here, the olecranon fossa and remainder of the posterior joint can be visualized and any loose bodies removed.

A simple but effective method to aid in visualization is to switch to a 70° arthroscope. The advantages of using a 70° arthroscope are that it can allow for complete visualization of the coronoid fossa and potential loose bodies in the anterior joint. It also allows for complete visualization of the posterolateral and posteromedial gutters, as well as the olecranon fossa and radiocapitellar joint in the posterior aspect of the elbow [18].

A grading system has been developed by Baumgarten, et al. to aid in decision-making during elbow arthroscopy. The grading is summarized in Table 3.1. The recommendation presented for Grade 1 lesions is either observation or arthroscopic drilling of the lesion. Grade 2 lesions were treated with debridement of the cartilage to healthy tissue. Grade 3 lesions were treated with loosening of the fragment to create a Grade 4 lesion, which was then resected. Grade 5 lesions were

Table 3.1 Classification system suggested by Baumgarten et al. [11]

Grade 1	Smooth but soft, ballotable articular cartilage
Grade 2	Fibrillations or fissuring of the articular cartilage
Grade 3	Exposed bone with a fixed osteochondral fragment
Grade 4	Loose but undisplaced fragment
Grade 5	Displaced fragment with resultant loose bodies

treated with a diligent search for the loose bodies. All lesions with exposed bone were also treated with abrasion chondroplasty. The results showed good results in short term follow up [11].

Postoperative management includes range of motion as tolerated following 2–3 days in a splint at 90°. Active and passive motion in physical therapy is started as soon as the splint is removed, and patients are permitted to return to normal activity as soon as they are comfortable.

3.6   Complications

The most worrisome complication associated with arthroscopy of the elbow is neurovascular injury. Neurological injury can occur to the radial nerve, posterior interosseous nerve and ulnar nerve. The radial nerve palsy is often transient and is thought to be associated with extravasation of fluid through the anterolateral portal [19]. Complete transection of the median and ulnar nerves has even been reported [20]. Using the portals described above can attenuate the risk of neurologic injury.

Other risks are associated with arthroscopy in general to include infection, persistent drainage and articular cartilage damage [6, 19].

3.7   Results

The results of treatment for OCD lesions of the elbow have been mixed. While most studies show good short term results, few long term studies exist [9–11, 21–26]. Results of arthroscopic debridement, drilling, microfracturing or fragment fixation have been shown to to provide a good return to sport level [23]. These techniques all share the advantage of being able to be performed arthroscopically. The small size of the elbow joint, lesion and overall size of the adolescent patient make an all-arthroscopic technique an attractive option. Although a more recent study has shown that while the return to sport may be high, the sport returned to may not necessarily be the sport that was being participated in at the time of injury [26].

A recently published study examining the short term clinical results and MRI findings after microfracture show encouraging results. The mean time to final clinical follow up was 42 months and the mean time to final radiographic follow up was 27 months. All of the patients were able to return to some form of sport, and all of the patients showed some MRI evidence of cartilage filling of the lesions [27].

Osteochondral autograft has also been shown to have good return to sport levels [23, 28, 29]. The advantage of using an osteochondral autograft is it is the only technique to reproduce hyaline cartilage at the defect site. The downside is potential donor site morbidity, as well as the need for greater exposure to the lesion. This can be particularly problematic in the elbow with associated small lesions.

References

1. Kusumi T, Ishibashi Y, Tsuda E, Kusumi A, Tanaka M, Sato F, Toh S, Kijima H (2006) Osteochondritis dissecans of the elbow: histopathological assessment of the articular cartilage and subchondral bone with emphasis on their damage and repair. Pathol Int 56(10):604–612. doi:10.1111/j.1440-1827.2006.02015.x
2. Mihara K, Tsutsui H, Nishinaka N, Yamaguchi K (2009) Nonoperative treatment for osteochondritis dissecans of the capitellum. Am J Sports Med 37(2):298–304. doi: 10.1177/0363546508324970
3. Takahara M, Mura N, Sasaki J, Harada M, Ogino T (2008) Classification, treatment, and outcome of osteochondritis dissecans of the humeral capitellum. Surgical technique. J Bone Joint Surg Am 90 Suppl 2 Pt 1:47–62. doi:10.2106/JBJS.G.01135
4. Takahara M, Ogino T, Fukushima S, Tsuchida H, Kaneda K (1999) Nonoperative treatment of osteochondritis dissecans of the humeral capitellum. Am J Sports Med 27(6):728–732
5. van den Ende KI, McIntosh AL, Adams JE, Steinmann SP (2011) Osteochondritis dissecans of the capitellum: a review of the literature and a distal ulnar portal. Arthroscopy: J Arthrosc Relat Surg: Official Publ Arthroscopy Assoc North Am Int Arthrosc Assoc 27(1):122–128. doi:10.1016/j.arthro.2010.08.008
6. Dodson CC, Nho SJ, Williams RJ 3rd, Altchek DW (2008) Elbow arthroscopy. J Am Acad Orthop Surg 16(10):574–585
7. Panner HJ (1929) A peculiar affection of the capitulum humeri, resembling calve-perthes disease of the hip. Acta Radiol 10(3):234–242
8. Pappas AM (1981) Osteochondrosis dissecans. Clin Orthop Relat Res 158:59–69
9. Ruch DS, Cory JW, Poehling GG (1998) The arthroscopic management of osteochondritis dissecans of the adolescent elbow. Arthroscopy: J Arthrosc Relat Surg: Official Publ Arthroscopy Assoc North Am Int Arthrosc Assoc 14(8):797–803
10. Baker CL 3rd, Romeo AA, Baker CL Jr (2010) Osteochondritis dissecans of the capitellum. Am J Sports Med 38(9):1917–1928. doi:10.1177/0363546509354969
11. Baumgarten TE, Andrews JR, Satterwhite YE (1998) The arthroscopic classification and treatment of osteochondritis dissecans of the capitellum. Am J Sports Med 26(4):520–523
12. De Smet AA, Ilahi OA, Graf BK (1996) Reassessment of the MR criteria for stability of osteochondritis dissecans in the knee and ankle. Skeletal Radiol 25(2):159–163
13. Dipaola JD, Nelson DW, Colville MR (1991) Characterizing osteochondral lesions by magnetic resonance imaging. Arthroscopy: J Arthrosc Relat Surg: Official Publ Arthroscopy Assoc North Am Int Arthrosc Assoc 7(1):101–104
14. Iwasaki N, Kamishima T, Kato H, Funakoshi T, Minami A (2012) A retrospective evaluation of magnetic resonance imaging effectiveness on capitellar osteochondritis dissecans among overhead athletes. Am J Sports Med 40(3):624–630. doi:10.1177/0363546511429258
15. Kijowski R, Blankenbaker DG, Shinki K, Fine JP, Graf BK, De Smet AA (2008) Juvenile versus adult osteochondritis dissecans of the knee: appropriate MR imaging criteria for instability. Radiology 248(2):571–578. doi:10.1148/radiol.2482071234

16. Shi LL, Bae DS, Kocher MS, Micheli LJ, Waters PM (2012) Contained versus uncontained lesions in juvenile elbow osteochondritis dissecans. J Pediatr Orthop 32(3):221–225. doi: 10.1097/BPO.0b013e31824afecf
17. Poehling GG, Whipple TL, Sisco L, Goldman B (1989) Elbow arthroscopy: a new technique. Arthroscopy: J Arthrosc Relat Surg: Official Publ Arthroscopy Assoc North Am Int Arthrosc Assoc 5(3):222–224
18. Bedi A, Dines J, Dines DM, Kelly BT, O'Brien SJ, Altchek DW, Allen AA (2010) Use of the 70° arthroscope for improved visualization with common arthroscopic procedures. Arthroscopy: J Arthrosc Relat Surg: Official Publ Arthroscopy Assoc North Am Int Arthrosc Assoc 26(12):1684–1696. doi:10.1016/j.arthro.2010.04.070
19. O'Driscoll SW, Morrey BF (1992) Arthroscopy of the elbow. Diagnostic and therapeutic benefits and hazards. J Bone Joint Surg Am 74 (1):84–94
20. Haapaniemi T, Berggren M, Adolfsson L (1999) Complete transection of the median and radial nerves during arthroscopic release of post-traumatic elbow contracture. Arthroscopy: J Arthrosc Relat Surg: Official Publ Arthroscopy Assoc North Am Int Arthrosc Assoc 15(7):784–787
21. Bauer M, Jonsson K, Josefsson PO, Linden B (1992) Osteochondritis dissecans of the elbow. A long-term follow-up study. Clin Orthop Relat Res 284:156–160
22. Bradley JP, Petrie RS (2001) Osteochondritis dissecans of the humeral capitellum. Diagnosis and treatment. Clin Sports Med 20(3):565–590
23. de Graaff F, Krijnen MR, Poolman RW, Willems WJ (2011) Arthroscopic surgery in athletes with osteochondritis dissecans of the elbow. Arthroscopy: J Arthrosc Relat Surg: Official Publ Arthroscopy Assoc North Am Int Arthrosc Assoc 27(7):986–993. doi: 10.1016/j.arthro.2011.01.002
24. Rahusen FT, Brinkman JM, Eygendaal D (2006) Results of arthroscopic debridement for osteochondritis dissecans of the elbow. Br J Sports Med 40(12):966–969. doi: 10.1136/bjsm.2006.030056
25. Schoch B, Wolf BR (2010) Osteochondritis dissecans of the capitellum: minimum 1-year follow-up after arthroscopic debridement. Arthroscopy: J Arthrosc Relat Surg: Official Publ Arthroscopy Assoc North Am Int Arthrosc Assoc 26(11):1469–1473. doi: 10.1016/j.arthro.2010.03.008
26. Tis JE, Edmonds EW, Bastrom T, Chambers HG (2012) Short-term results of arthroscopic treatment of osteochondritis dissecans in skeletally immature patients. J Pediatr Orthop 32(3):226–231. doi:10.1097/BPO.0b013e31824afeb8
27. Wulf CA, Stone RM, Giveans MR, Lervick GN (2012) Magnetic resonance imaging after arthroscopic microfracture of capitellar osteochondritis dissecans. Am J Sports Med. doi: 10.1177/0363546512458765
28. Iwasaki N, Kato H, Ishikawa J, Masuko T, Funakoshi T, Minami A (2009) Autologous osteochondral mosaicplasty for osteochondritis dissecans of the elbow in teenage athletes. J Bone Joint Surg Am 91(10):2359–2366. doi:10.2106/JBJS.H.01266
29. Yamamoto Y, Ishibashi Y, Tsuda E, Sato H, Toh S (2006) Osteochondral autograft transplantation for osteochondritis dissecans of the elbow in juvenile baseball players: minimum 2-year follow-up. Am J Sports Med 34(5):714–720. doi:10.1177/03635465 05282620

Arthroscopic Treatment of Lateral Epicondylitis

4

Champ L. Baker Jr and Champ L. Baker III

4.1 Introduction

Surgical treatment is indicated for patients with recalcitrant symptoms of lateral epicondylitis or lateral elbow pain; however, the success of any surgical technique depends on proper patient selection, identification of the pathology, and complete resection of the pathologic tendinosis tissue. Arthroscopic treatment is a relatively new concept of managing these symptoms with techniques that have advanced over the last 20 years. In addition to the other advantages of arthroscopy the ability to resect the pathologic tendinosis tissue of the extensor carpi radialis brevis (ECRB) origin through an inside–out approach is foremost. Because the capsule closely adheres to the ECRB, once it is débrided, the tendon's pathologic tissue can be easily visualized and treated. Another advantage of the arthroscopic technique is the surgeon's ability to address coexistent intra-articular pathology, such as radiocapitellar joint arthritis, synovitis, or as is often the case, a thickened annular ligament, or plica of the elbow. These conditions can mimic epicondylitis, and surgical treatment through an open approach without intra-articular evaluation of the joint can cause the surgeon to miss the true or additional cause of lateral elbow pain.

Three published papers are helpful in demonstrating the arthroscopic technique and its safety and reliability [1–3]. In 1999, Kuklo et al. [1] published the findings of their cadaveric dissection of 10 upper extremities to determine the safety of the procedure. The investigators completed an arthroscopic visualization of the extensor tendon and resection of the ECRB tendon. Following this, they dissected the elbow to examine the distance of the cannula from the radial, median, ulnar, lateral antebrachial, and posterior antebrachial nerves, and the brachial artery, and

C. L. Baker Jr (✉) · C. L. Baker III
The Hughston Clinic, 6262 Veterans Parkway, Columbus, GA 31909, USA
e-mail: cbaker@hughston.com

L. A. Pederzini (ed.), *Elbow Arthroscopy*,
DOI: 10.1007/978-3-642-38103-4_4, © ISAKOS 2013

the ulnar collateral ligament. There was no direct laceration of the neurovascular structures. The ulnar collateral ligament was not destabilized or harmed and the resection of the ECRB was demonstrated. They concluded that it was a safe, reliable, and reproducible technique.

In 2006, Cummins [2] published a report on the results of this arthroscopic procedure performed on case series of 18 patients. In his study, patients underwent arthroscopic debridement for chronic lateral epicondylitis. The arthroscopic procedure was followed by a traditional open procedure for gross and histological analysis. He found that although not all patients had complete resection of the tendinopathy, 8 of the 18 had no gross evidence of residual tendinopathy after arthroscopic debridement. Poorer outcomes were identified in the 10 who had residual histologic evidence of tendinopathy. They concluded arthroscopic debridement and resection for ECRB arthroscopically could be performed and all pathological tissue could be removed, although they warned it did not happen in every case.

In the third study published in 2008, Cohen et al. [3] used cadaveric specimens to look at the anatomic relationships of the extensor tendon origin and the implications of arthroscopic treatment. They concluded the following: (1) the elbow capsule must be resected, (2) the bony origin of the ECRB was reliably identified beneath the distal-most aspect of the supracondylar ridge of the humerus, and (3) the tendinous origin of the ECRB must be released from the top of the capitellum to the midline of the radiocapitellar joint. In all 10 specimens, they found a safe and complete arthroscopic release was completed.

The 3 previously cited published studies form the basis of opinion that arthroscopic resection of the ECRB is reproducible and is safe using appropriate guidelines, and arthroscopic removal of all pathologic tissue is possible.

4.2   Surgical Technique

Elbow arthroscopy can be performed with the patient in the supine, prone, or lateral decubitus position. The technique with the patient in either the prone or lateral decubitus position is essentially the same. Two primary portals are used: the proximal medial is used for visualization, and the proximal lateral is used for operative procedures. Occasionally, a secondary superolateral portal may be needed for retraction. The pathoanatomy of the ECRB is identified arthroscopically, and using the classification system of Baker et al. [4], changes in the joint are classified as a type I lesion (intact capsule), a type II lesion (linear capsular tear), or a type III lesion (complete capsular tear) (Fig. 4.1). We also look for a thickened annular ligament or synovial fringe, as described by Mullett et al. [5]. Once the pathoanatomy has been identified, the procedure is straightforward.

With the patient under general or block anesthesia, the elbow is prepared and draped. Landmarks are identified and the medial epicondyle, lateral epicondyle, olecranon tip, radial head, and the ulnar nerve are outlined (Fig. 4.2). The joint is

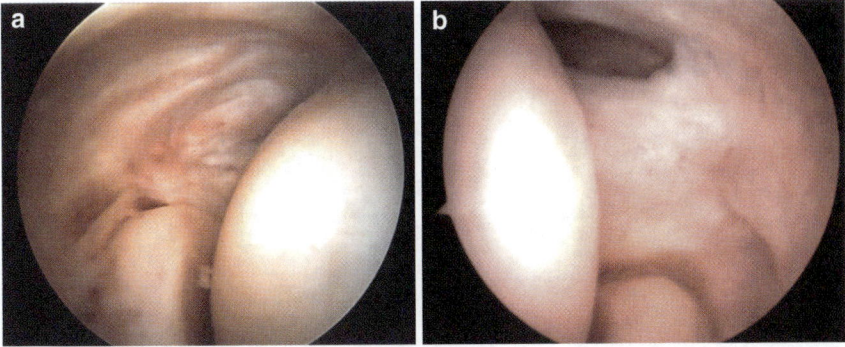

Fig. 4.1 Type II lesion (**a**) with partial tear of the capsule in a *right* elbow. Type III lesion (**b**) with complete rupture of the capsule in a *left* elbow

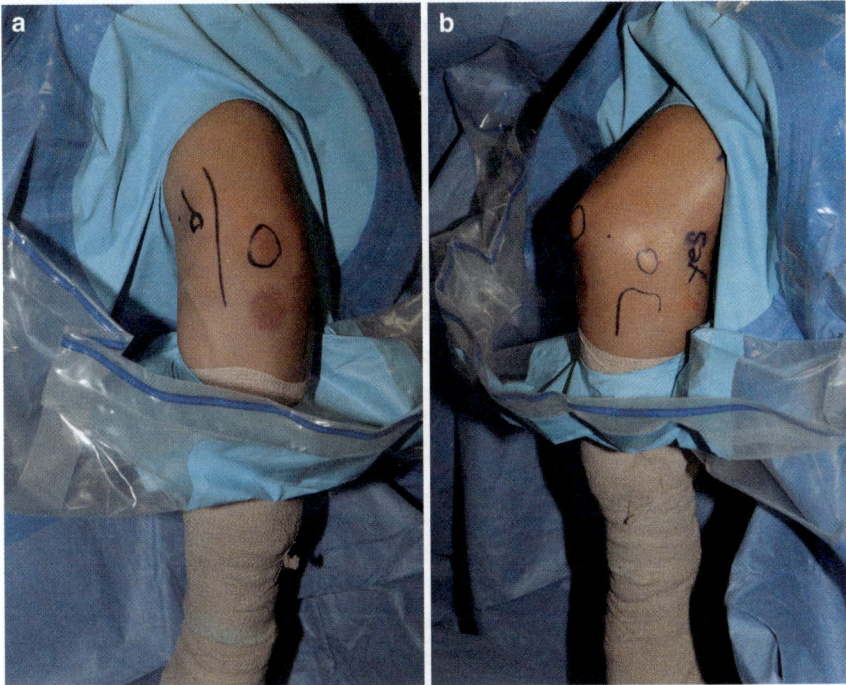

Fig. 4.2 **a** Landmarks outlined include medial epicondyle and intermuscular septum, ulnar nerve, and olecranon tip, and **b** the lateral epicondyle, and radial head

distended through a direct lateral portal with approximately 20 mL of fluid (Fig. 4.3). Distention of the anterior capsule pushes the neurovascular structures away from the joint and help to protect them from injury. The procedure is done under tourniquet control.

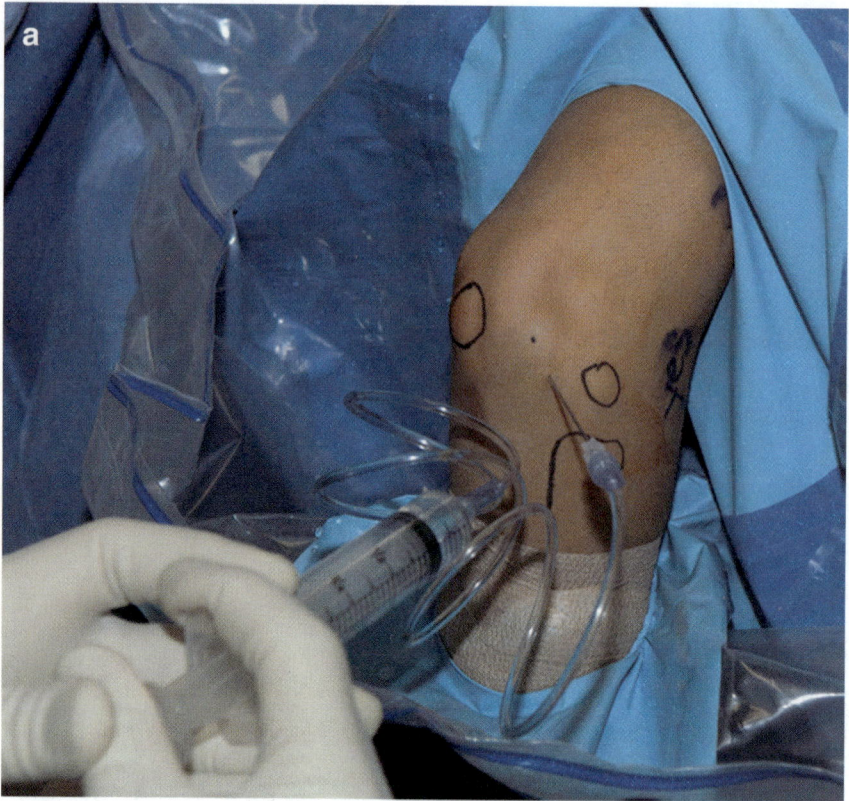

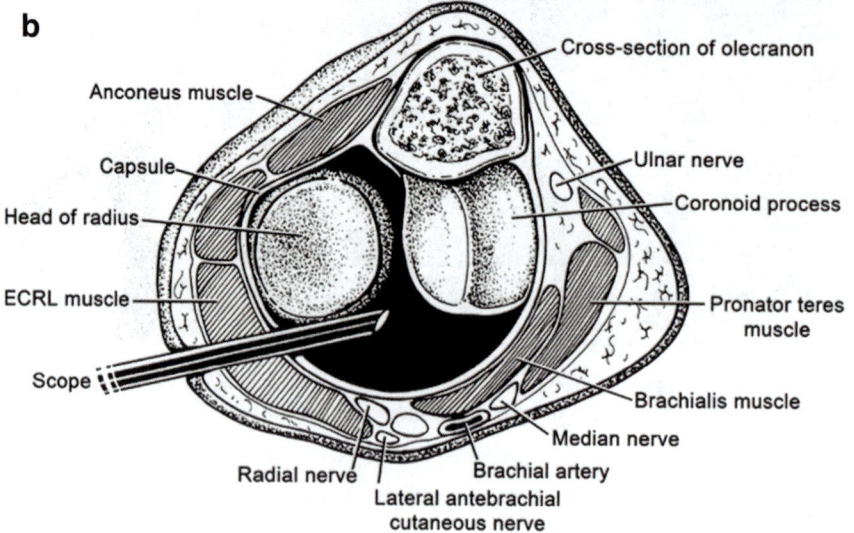

Fig. 4.3 **a** To distend the joint and displace the neurovascular structures anteriorly, 20–25 mL of fluid are injected through the lateral soft spot. **b** Distended joint with the arthroscope in a lateral portal showing proximity to neurovascular structures. *ECRL* extensor carpi radialis longus

Fig. 4.4 Relationship of the proximal medial portal to surrounding neurovascular structures

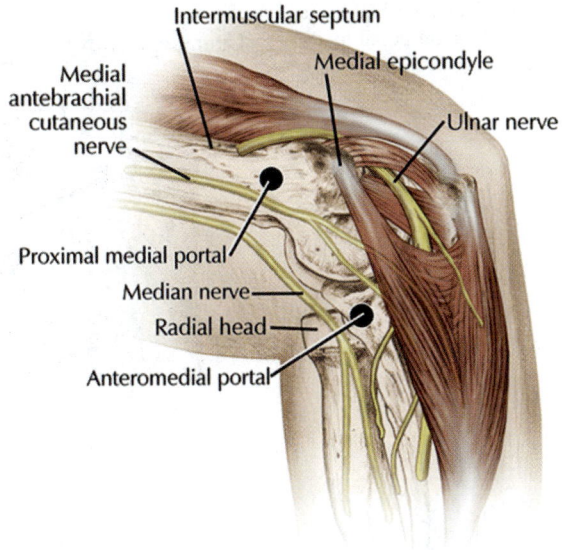

The nick-and-spread technique is used to create a **proximal medial** portal 2 cm proximal to the medial epicondyle and superior to the intermuscular septum (Fig. 4.4). An incision is made in the skin, a hemostat is used to spread the fascia, and an arthroscopic trocar is inserted and aimed toward the center of the joint. Once the portal is established, a pop can be felt as the trocar enters the capsule and joint. When fluid expressed through the cannula confirms entrance into the joint, the arthroscope is inserted.

We first visualize the radiocapitellar joint to identify pathology. Using an outside-in technique, a needle is used to localize insertion of a second proximal anterolateral portal cannula approximately 2 cm proximal and 1 cm anterior to the lateral epicondyle (Fig. 4.5). Initially, the capsule is débrided with a shaver. If necessary, a synovectomy or synovial fringe excision can also be performed with the shaver at this time. My preference is to use a monopolar radiofrequency probe for resection of tissue because it is malleable and can be bent to fit the contours of the elbow. It is sometimes difficult to gain initial purchase on the tendon with hand instruments and shavers. I have, by and large, abandoned them for radiofrequency probes, although hand instruments can be used to resect the tendon.

I use the 4-step technique described by Lattermann et al. [6] for release of the ECRB. The technique involves partial resection of the capsule, resection of the ECRB proximal and posterior to the extensor carpi radialis longus (ECRL), and resection anterior to the lateral collateral ligament and decortication of the origin of the ECRB. Once the capsule is released, the ECRB tendon is exposed. The tendon is the tissue lying between the lateral epicondyle and the underlying muscle belly of the extensor digitorum communis (EDC). We release proximal to the supracondylar

Fig. 4.5 Relationship of the proximal lateral portal to surrounding neurovascular structures

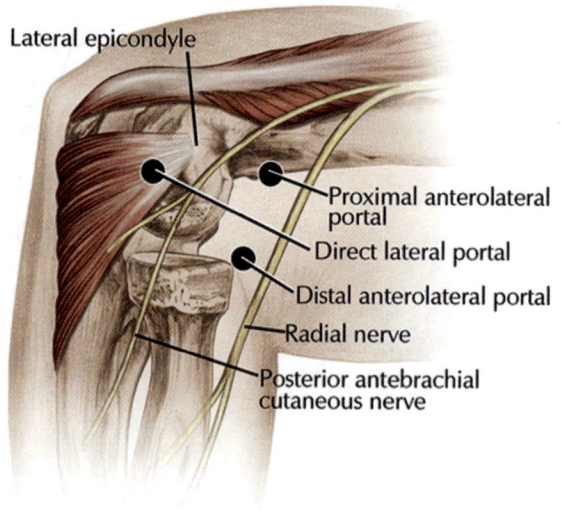

Lateral epicondyle

Proximal anterolateral portal

Direct lateral portal

Distal anterolateral portal

Radial nerve

Posterior antebrachial cutaneous nerve

ridge of the humerus and distal from the top of the capitellum to the midline of the radiocapitellar joint. In a 2003 publication by Smith et al. [7], we were alerted to the position of the lateral collateral ligament in relation to the radial head and capitellum. Damage to the ligament is avoided as long as the surgeon stays anterior to the radial head. In my patients, I never go inferior to the radial head and have had no instance of iatrogenic injury to the collateral ligament. Once the resection is complete, the surgeon can elect to decorticate the origin of the ECRB off the lateral epicondyle or can leave it alone. Initially, we used a burr to débride this area as is normally done in open surgery treatment. We theorized that it would promote bleeding and healing in the area for reattachment of the longus. In my experience, this step is not needed to get a good result, and there is some concern that a new trigger point for pain would develop where the bone was decorticated.

Of course, the arthroscopic procedure should include a complete evaluation of the anterior capsule. The surgeon can switch portals to look from the lateral across to the medial aspect for loose bodies or involvement of the coronoid trochlear articulation. The posterior compartment can be visualized at this time, and if there is a suggestion of a posterior radiocapitellar plica or posterior soft tissue impingement, debridement can be carried out if indicated.

At completion, the wound is closed with interrupted nylon ligature and a compressive wrap is applied. A local anesthetic can be injected into the portals for postoperative pain relief. However, a local anesthetic injected through the medial portal could affect the status of the ulnar nerve. The patient's arm is placed in a sling for comfort. Patients are encouraged to remove the sling as quickly as tolerated and work on active and passive exercises, working toward full extension with passive extension of the digits. All patients received a course of therapy with instructions on home exercise programs.

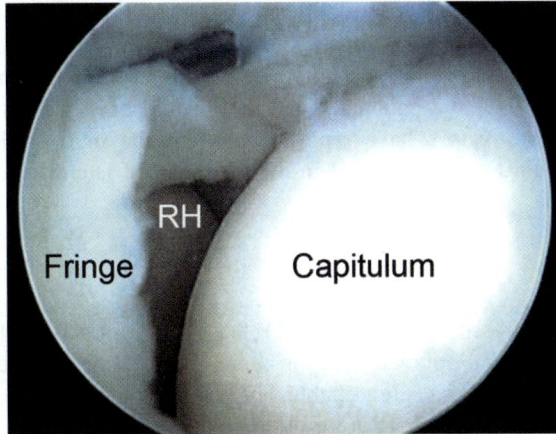

Fig. 4.6 Arthroscopic view of a lateral plica band (synovial fringe) of the capsule. *RH* radial head

A follow-up visit is usually scheduled 5–7 days after surgery for suture removal and examination of the operative sites. Patients progress in their rehabilitation depending on their symptoms and their sport or occupation. Often, the patient can return to work the next day. Return to a sport may take a little longer, and the return to a strenuous racquet-type sport can take from 8 to 12 weeks until full strength is achieved.

Lateral plica. Some patients have typical lateral elbow pain and a click with pronation and supination of the radiocapitellar joint without the classic findings of pain over the ECRB and pain on passive volar flexion or dorsiflexion against resistance of the wrist. These patients may also have some pain on forced extension. They may fall into the subgroup of patients with a lateral plica band or thickened annular ligament as described by Mullet et al. [5]. At arthroscopy, a cord-like band of the capsule that impinges and subluxates can often be seen (Fig. 4.6). A classification system based on the relationship of the capsular fold to the radial head was described by Mullett et al. [5]: Type 1, the radial head is completely disclosed; Type 2, there is partial coverage of the radial head by the capsuloligamentous complex without interposition into the joint; Type 3, there is subluxation of the capsular edge into the joint; and Type 4, the radial head is completely obscured throughout the range of motion. Antuna and O'Driscoll [8] also studied plicae, or hypertrophic synovial folds, and stated, "The presence of synovial plicae in the radiocapitellar joint must be considered in the differential diagnosis of painful snapping elbow. Arthroscopy confirms the diagnosis and allows excision of the plica."

4.3 Results

Numerous articles in the literature report the results of arthroscopic treatment of lateral epicondylitis. We published the 2-year results in 42 patients treated with arthroscopic lateral release in 2000 [4] and followed that in 2008 [9] with a

10-year follow-up report on 30 of our original patients. We found that the mean pain score at rest in these patients was 0 on a scale of 0 (no pain) to 10 (severe pain). No patients required further surgery or repeat injections. When interviewed, 93 % of the patients stated they would have the surgery again, if needed. Other investigators have reported good results in over 90 % of patients undergoing arthroscopic resection in the treatment of lateral epicondylitis [6, 10].

4.4   Conclusion

Arthroscopic resection and release of the ECRB tendinous origin in the treatment of lateral epicondylitis for lateral elbow pain has been demonstrated in cadaveric studies to be safe, reliable, and reproducible. In clinical studies, the procedure has demonstrated efficacy, a low complication rate, and a quick return to work with results that last over a long period of time. Results are comparable to or better than those for traditional open methods.

References

1. Kuklo TR, Taylor KF, Murphy KP et al (1999) Arthroscopic release for lateral epicondylitis: a cadaveric model. Arthroscopy 15(3):259–264
2. Cummins CA (2006) Lateral epicondylitis: in vivo assessment of arthroscopic debridement and correlation with patient outcomes. Am J Sports Med 34(9):1486–1491
3. Cohen MS, Romeo AA, Hennigan SP (2008) Lateral epicondylitis: anatomic relationships of the extensor tendon origins and implications for arthroscopic treatment. J Shoulder Elbow Surg 17(6):954–960
4. Baker CL, Murphy KP, Gottlob CA (2000) Arthroscopic classification and treatment of lateral epicondylitis: two-year clinical results. J Shoulder Elbow Surg 9(6):475–482
5. Mullett H, Sprague M, Brown G (2005) Arthroscopic treatment of lateral epicondylitis: clinical and cadaveric studies. Clin Orthop Relat Res 439:123–128
6. Lattermann C, Romeo AA, Anbari A (2010) Arthroscopic debridement of the extensor carpi radialis brevis for recalcitrant lateral epicondylitis. J Shoulder Elbow Surg 19(5):651–656
7. Smith AM, Castle JA, Ruch DS (2003) Arthroscopic resection of the common extensor origin: anatomic considerations. J Shoulder Elbow Surg 12(4):375–379
8. Antuna SA, O'Driscoll SW (2001) Snapping plicae associated with radiocapitellar chondromalacia. Arthroscopy 17(5):491–495
9. Baker CL Jr, Baker CL 3rd (2008) Long-term follow-up of arthroscopic treatment of lateral epicondylitis. Am J Sports Med 36(2):254–260
10. Savoie FH, VanSice W, O'Brien MJ (2010) Arthroscopic tennis elbow release. J Shoulder Elbow Surg 19(2 Suppl):31–36

Elbow Arthroscopy in Stiff Elbow

5

Luigi Pederzini, Massimo Tosi, Mauro Prandini and Fabio Nicoletta

5.1 Introduction

Arthroscopy is increasingly used to diagnose and treat elbow pathologies although the elbow has always been considered a difficult joint to be endoscopically explored. Arthroscopy knowledge increase and technology breakthrough in the last few years have allowed a standardisation of techniques and a better definition of indications. In the 1980s Andrews and Carson [1], Hempfling [2] and Lindelfeld [3] published the first indications, techniques and notions on elbow arthroscopy. In 1981, on the basis of their observations, Morrey et al. [4] determined that the elbow functional motion ranged from 30 to 130° of flexion; however, a lot of daily activities performed at work or while doing physical exercise require an extension above 30°. As a matter of fact, for sportsmen and manual workers even a small decrease in ROM, together with slight symptoms of pain and inability to perform specific tasks, can be unacceptable and, hence, interfere with their daily work or sport activities. For this reason, there has been an extension of indications concerning stiff elbows treatment. In 1992 O'Driscoll and Morrey [5] presented 72 cases of elbow arthroscopy and in 2001 they published a review of 473 cases in which they analysed the complications related to this procedure [6]. The previous year, Reddy et al. [7] had published a review of 172 cases in which patients had undergone arthroscopic elbow surgery with a 7-year-follow up. The list of indications for elbow arthroscopy has grown over the past years and today it includes osteochondritis dissecans (OCD), plica syndrome, sinoviectomy in R.A. and other synovitis, lateral epicondilitis, loose bodies removal [8–12], stiff elbows related to degenerative or post-traumatic causes [13–16]. Recently, Conso [17] as well as

L. Pederzini (✉) · M. Tosi · M. Prandini · F. Nicoletta
Department of Othopaedic, Othopaedic Sassuolo Hospital, Street saragozza 130, 41100 Modena, Italy
e-mail: gigiped@hotmail.com

L. A. Pederzini (ed.), *Elbow Arthroscopy*,
DOI: 10.1007/978-3-642-38103-4_5, © ISAKOS 2013

43

Shubert [18] and Salini [19] have published the results obtained by comparing respectively 32, 24 and 15 arthroscopic cases presenting a moderate stiffness of the elbow and other pathologies, with those obtained with open techniques. There are several studies regarding this subject in literature, but all of them are based on a small number of patients with a variety of pathologies treated with different surgical techniques [20–28].

5.2   Causes and Indications

While postraumatic stiff elbow is strictly connected to a recent trauma (one year), degenerative stiff elbow pictures can be determined by overuse syndromes, primary ostheoartritic changes or sequelae of not recent (more than one year) traumatic event. Every single decrease of the elbow ROM can be considered as a stiff elbow depending from the work, sport activity and functional request of the patient. Clinical evaluation must consider sex, dominant arm, etiopathogenesis, pre-operative MEPI (Pain, ROM, balance and function), radiological and clinical findings. After considering 6 months-failure of conservative treatment (mobilisation, splinting and physical therapy), intact articular space, absence or mild anatomical incongruency, ROM reduction, sport and occupation related disability, a patient can be candidate for an arthroscopic arthrolisis. On the other hand arthroscopic technique can be useful in association with open surgery in order to avoid large surgical approaches. Sometimes removal of a columnar plate or screws can be associated with an arthroscopic arthrolisis.

Many traumatic events like fracture of the olecranon, radial head, coronoid, fracture dislocation, dislocations determine stiffness in a late follow up and, respecting the previous indications, can be treated arthroscopically.

Degenerative elbows can occur in "overuse syndromes" in manual workers and sportsmen in which the continuous training or heavy work can produce early degeneration of the joint [28]. Javelin, baseball, boxeurs, weight lifters, tennis player often present typical degenerative elbows.

Again reumathoid arthritis (early stages) and osteochondropaties can also be considered candidate for an arthroscopic treatment.

Presence of osteophites, sinovitis, loose bodies is also an anatomo pathological finding in course of a previous not recent trauma (radial head fracture, coronoid fracture etc.) in which the altered joint mechanism, allows to develop an early degenerative picture.

We exclude from the arthroscopic procedure all muscle spasticity, cerebral paralysis, burns, previous surgeries leading to anatomical alterations, heterotopic ossifications, ossificans myositis, algodystrophy, articular instability, anatomic incongruence and infections related stiffness cases.

5.3 Surgical Technique in Stiff Elbow

Anaesthetist identifies nerve trunks by applying electro stimulation and places a catether without injecting the anaesthetic. Patients then undergo general anaesthesia. When they wake up, only after a neurological evaluation, peripheral block is performed. After the induction of anaesthesia, ROM is carefully assessed and a complete ligamentous balancing is carried out. The tourniquet is inflated to 250 mmHg. The patient is then placed prone, with the shoulder abducted 90°, the elbow flexed to 90° and the arm held up by an arm holder secured to the operating table. Sterile field is set up and elbow joint landmarks are drawn by a dermographic pen (medial and lateral epycondile, ulnar nerve, radial head, posterior soft spot). Soft spot posterior portals, supero-antero medial and supero-antero lateral portals are marked (Fig. 5.1). Ulnar nerve neurolysis has always been performed by making a 2 cm skin incision, except in full ROM cases (full ROM painful elbows, occasionally decreased ROM). An 18-gauge needle is inserted in the elbow through the "soft-spot" in the middle of the triangular area delimited by the epicondyle, the radial head and the olecranon, while the joint is distended by injecting 20 ml of N-Saline solution to introduce the trocar while shifting neurovascular anterior structures away. 5 portals, 3 posterior and 2 anterior, are always used. After the incision is made, soft tissues are retracted by using a fine haemostat. Posterior compartment arthroscopy is firstly performed by introducing a 4, 5 mm 30° arthroscope through the posterolateral portal (soft spot). Then a second portal is established, 1, 5 cm proximal to the latter. These two portals allow to use the scope and the shaver at the same level of the posterior portion of the radial head. Joint distension is achieved by a pump set at 35–50 mmHg. Once we get a good and complete view of the proximal radio-ulnar joint (posteriorly), a

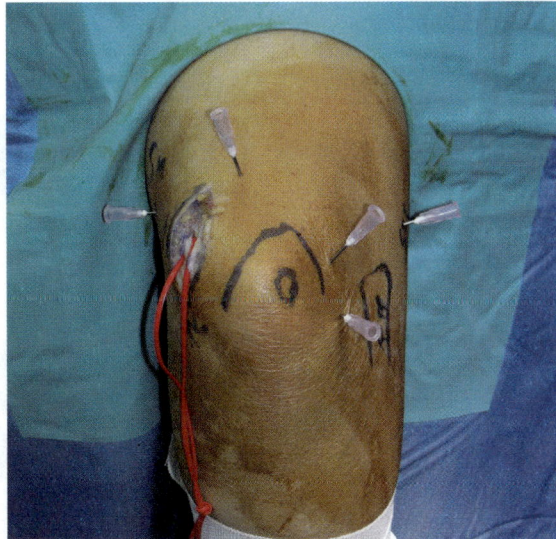

Fig. 5.1 Pink needles show posterior portals and supero medial and supero lateral anterior portals. The ulnar nerve is isolated

third posterior portal is placed in the olecranon fossa, close to the triceps medial border and oriented 2–3 cm proximal to the olecranon tip. A complete olecranon fossa and its lateral wall debridement can be performed as well as, if present, a lateral olecranon and humerus loose bodies removal to allow a better sliding of the articular surfaces. We use a different approach related to osteophytes dimension and ulnar nerve presence on the medial side. After inserting the arthroscope through the most proximal portal, we evaluate osteophytes dimensions; if they are small we protect the ulnar nerve by positioning a retractor in an accessory portal slightly posterior to the ulnar nerve (Fig. 5.2), and we resect the ostheophytes arthroscopically. If they are large, we prefer to remove the ostheophytes by performing a small arthrotomy at the end of the procedure, thus avoiding fluid extravasation during arthroscopy. The medial approach is always used after ulnar nerve neurolysis, which is the first surgical step of the procedure. This is necessary to prevent the overstretching of the nerve testing flexion and extension during elbow arthroscopy. The scope is then introduced in the anterior compartment through the supero-antero medial portal, 2 cm proximal and 1 cm anterior to the epitrochlea. The medial approach is preferable because it allows to locate the ulnar nerve by palpation, which is not possible on the lateral side. The antero-lateral portal is created using an inside-out technique and placing a Wissinger rod 2 cm proximal and 1 cm anterior to the lateral epicondyle. A plastic cannula is introduced on the rod and, subsequently after having the rod removed, a shaver can be positioned and the anterior debridement carried out (removal of loose bodies, anterior ostheophytes and sinoviectomy). In several cases, in presence of thick capsule (post-traumatic causes), an anterior capsulectomy may be required (Fig. 5.3). We start trimming the proximal humeral capsule by a shaver, but the real anterior capsulectomy is performed by a basket forceps, at about 1 cm proximally to the apex of the coronoid, firstly in a lateral-medial and then in a medial–lateral direction. After arthroscopy, ROM is assessed. One or two suction drainages are positioned into the joint, arthroscopic accesses are sutured and a

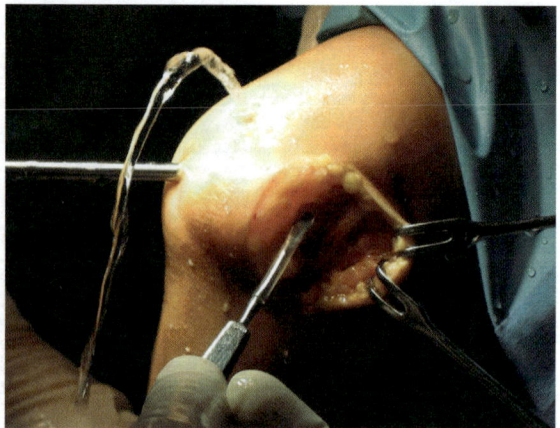

Fig. 5.2 Arthroscope in postero lateral inferior portal, fluid from postero lateral middle portal, a retractor can be indroduced in the postero medial accessory portal (in the subcutaneous tissue) posterior to the ulnar nerve

Fig. 5.3 Anterior
capsulectomy is performed.
View of anterior
compartment, residual
capsule and brachialis muscle

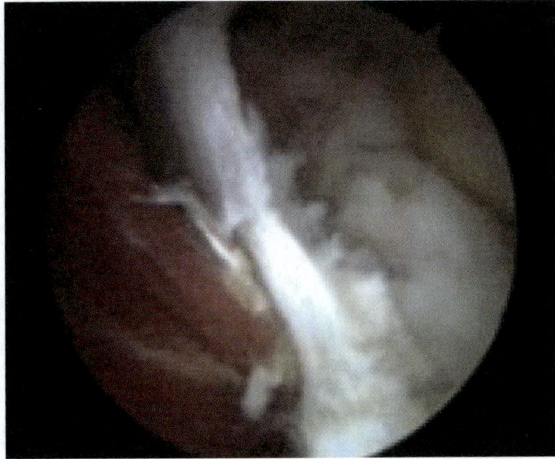

splint holding the joint in full extension is applied to correct the articular loss of
extension. On post-op day 1, patients start a 20 min Continuous Passive Motion
(CPM) 4 times a day, together with an assisted physiokinesis therapy, at least
60 min per day. On day 2 they start a self-assisted active and passive mobilisation
in flexion–extension. On day 3 drains are removed and we continue with the
rehabilitative program. Indometacine 50 mg 3 times per day is somministrated for
15 days. At the time of discharge from the hospital, patients are taught the exercises they need to practice at home. They continue the same programme with a
therapist for 3 months.

5.4 Surgical Technique in Radial Head Resection and Post Radial Head Resection

In case of not correct fixation of a radial head fracture or in case of vitious
consolidation of a radial head fracture we can observe a stiff elbow (decreased
flexion–extension and prono-supination) mainly due to a radial head problems
(nonunion, incongruency with increased diameter). Xray and 3D CT scan confirmed the lesion and indicate radial head resection.

Arthroscopic resection of the radial head (Figs. 5.4, 5.5, 5.6 and 5.7) can be
performed using 3 posterior portals and 2 anterior portals. After the identification
of the radial head and its posterior border the resection is carried out beginning
from the posterior margin with a small burr. This often offers us the opportunity to
resect the main part of the abnormal radial head and finishing the procedure from
the anterior approaches in order to avoid that some small bony particles left in the
joint can irritate the sinovium. During the procedure pronation and supination can
facilitate the resection. Occasionally screws for the previous fixation can be
removed. A thorough washing out is necessary at the end of the procedure. In few

Fig. 5.4 Pre-op x ray show a non union of the radial head with screws not fixing the fracture

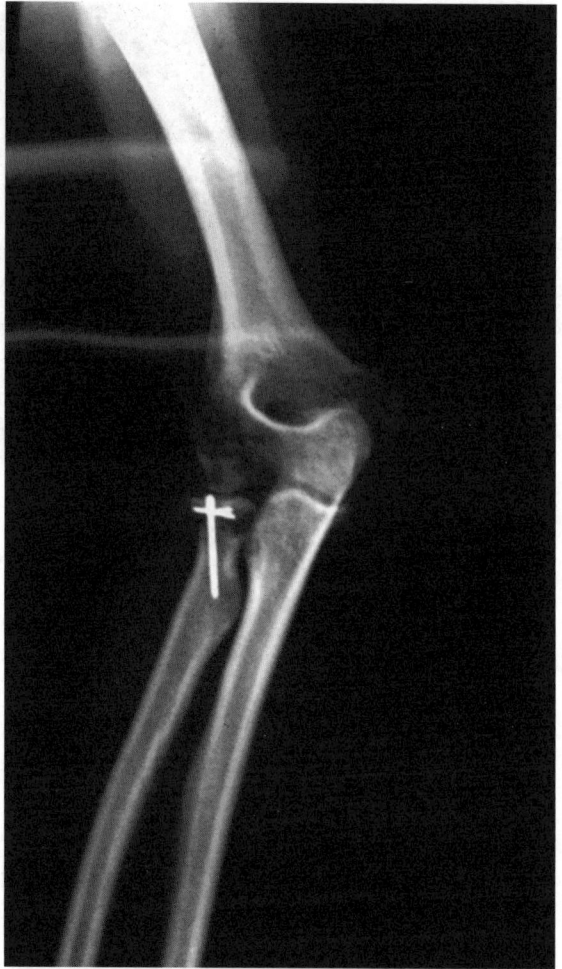

Fig. 5.5 Arthroscopic removal of the screws

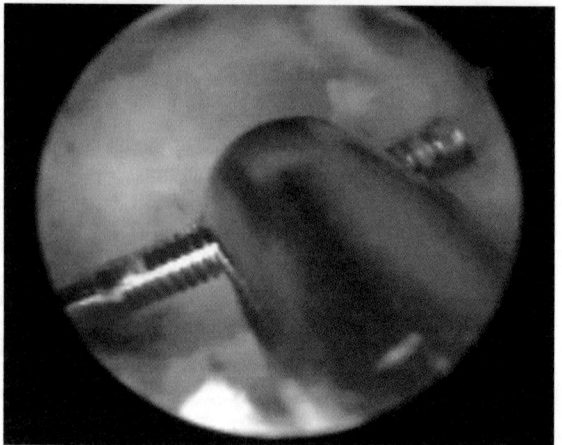

Fig. 5.6 Residual radius
after the resection

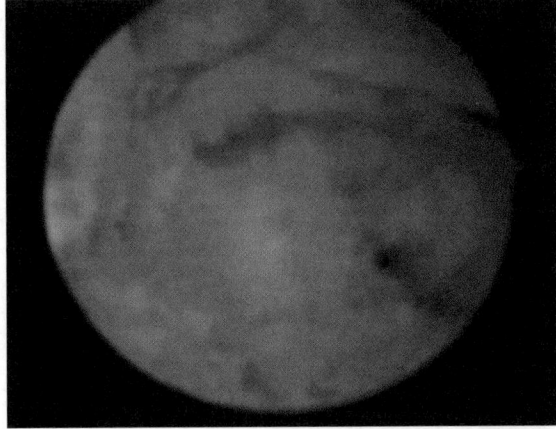

Fig. 5.7 post-op x rays show
the amount of the resection

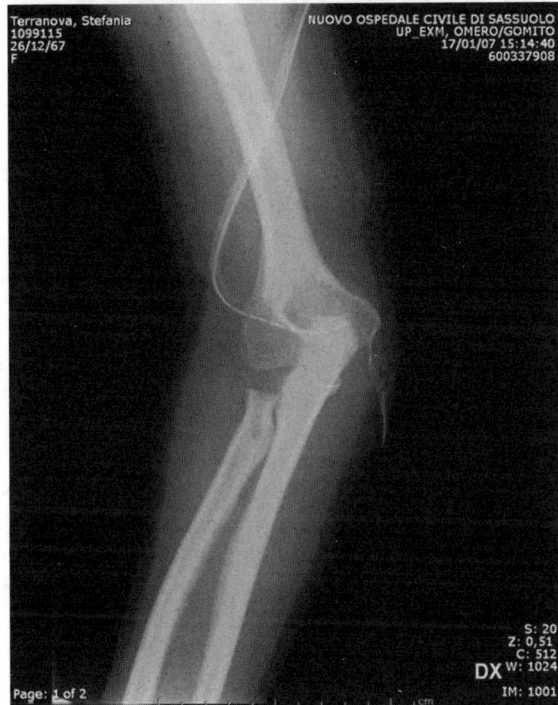

cases we performed arthroscopic arthrolisis after a previous radial head resection
with residual lock of prono supination probably due to a too limited resection and
fibrosis. In these cases a complete thick white fibrous tissue was found and
resected in between radial head and capitulum humeri then a more adequate bony
resection was carried out. In this case after to complete the posterior fossa

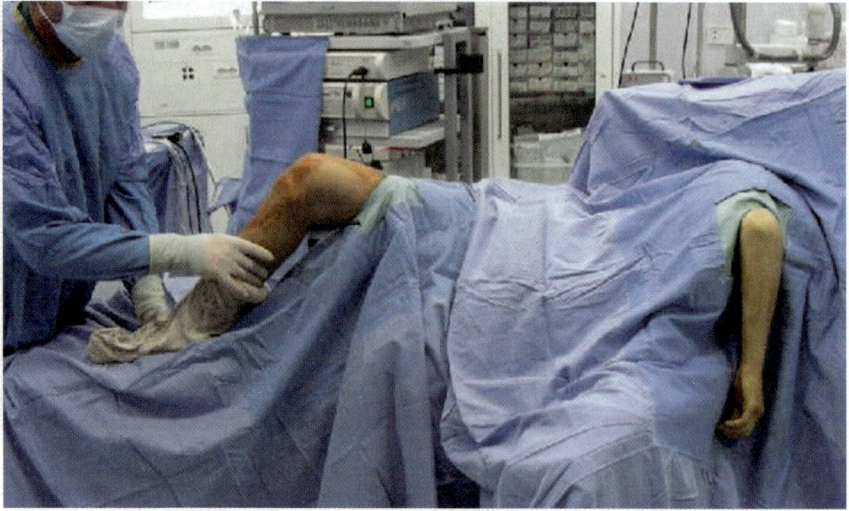

Fig. 5.8 Patient on lateral decubitus. Extrarotation of the hip allows to perform knee arthroscopy in order to take a graft from lateral troclea

debridement the antero lateral portal was indicated by a needle positioned in the space left from the removed radial head after the initial posterior debridement.

5.5 Surgical Technique in OCD

OCD can be a cause of painfull elbow with limited ROM. These young patients, usually athletes complaining pain and disfunction, limit their activity becoming unable to participate in sport.

Frequently located in the posterior part of the capitulum at 90° of flexion a complete detachment of the bone plug can occurred. Removal of the bone plug and microfracture is mandatory in order to eliminate catching and popping while it is still controversial the possibility to bone graft the lesion.

In some cases we performed an arthroscopic mosaic plasty taking the graft from the omolateral knee putting the patient in lateral decubitus and extra rotating the hip performing knee arthroscopy (Fig. 5.8). The 6.5 mm cylinder graft token from the lateral knee troclea was inserted in the elbow lesioned area carefully checking the angle of the drilling and of the insertion of the bony-cartilagineous cylinder. Arthroscopically the perpendicular insertion of the cylinder allows a complete coverage of the OCD area (Fig. 5.9 and 5.10). A 4 months later MRI (Fig. 5.11) shows a nice bone incorporation of the graft. Post-operatively the CPM started in day 2 and passive exercises in day 4. Patients were back to normal activity in 4 months.

Fig. 5.9 Dedicated
instrument to fill the lesioned
area with a knee graft

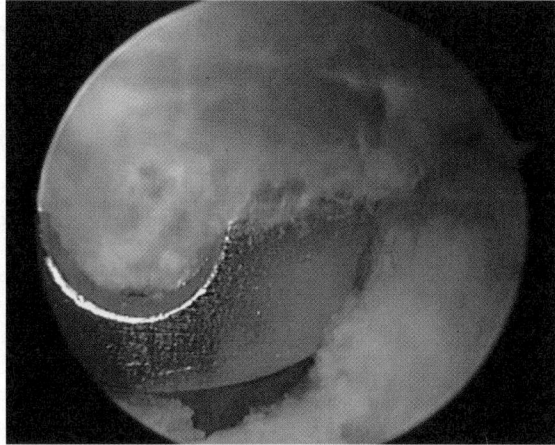

Fig. 5.10 Graft positioned
at the level of the cortical
bone

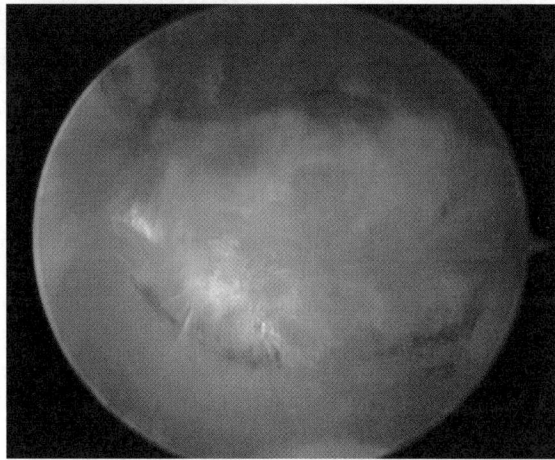

5.6   Rehabilitation Protocol

On day 1 after surgery, our rehabilitation protocol begins with a very slow CPM, 4 times a day for 40 min with the help of 2 suction drains and a perinervous anaesthetic catheter. On day 2, CPM 4 times a day for 40 min, plus 60 min of physiokinesitherapy and self active movements 4 times a day for 30 min. The third day starts with catheter removal and continues with CPM, FKT and self active movements. On day 4, the drains are removed and CPM, FKT and self active movements continue. On day 5, once discharged, the patient goes back home with a 20 days long re-educational program combined with indomethacin for 15 days. The splint is removed after 20 days. After 1 month patients get their first follow-up visit and rehabilitative program continues for 3–5 months.

Fig. 5.11 4 months MRI shows a perfect bone incorporation of the graft

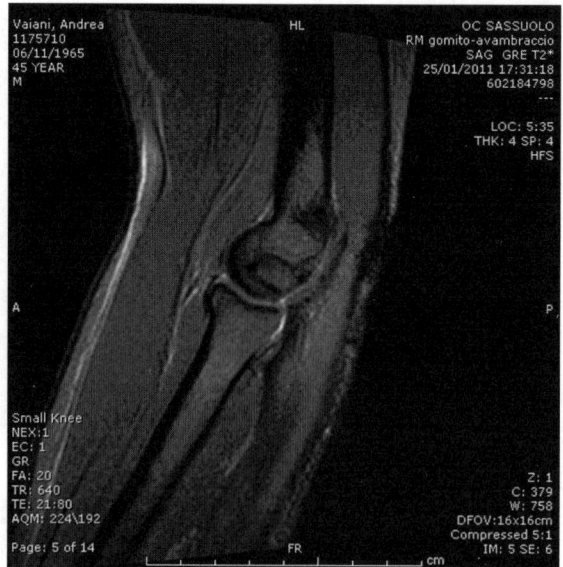

5.7   Discussion

In the last 15 years, elbow arthroscopy has been studied by different authors to reduce frequent complications described in previous authors' publications [29]. Anaesthesia and peripheral analgesic blocks are fundamental in order to assess potential neurological complications in the operating room and intervene if necessary. The use of different portals, the ulnar nerve isolation, the use of arthroscopic retractors and the avoidance of an excessive intraarticular joint pressure, are all fundamental elements for an accurate elbow arthroscopy. In other words it is important to achieve a clear arthroscopic vision, avoiding nerves and vessels injuries risks. Once established this, it will be easier to understand pathologies and their treatments. Post-traumatic and degenerative arthroscopic cases have different features. In post-traumatic cases the articular space is smaller, fibrosis is higher and capsule consistency, when removed by basket forceps, is stronger. In degenerative cases, articular space is larger, fibrosis is lower and capsule consistency weaker. Indications for stiffness arthroscopic treatment are still, in many cases, surgeon dependant. A more advanced learning curve guarantees a wider possibility to address post-traumatic pathologies and degenerative cases. Otherwise, the patient may be exposed to partial outcomes and/or complications.

In 2000 Reddy et al. presented a review of a large number of patients operated by several different surgeons, in different decubitus and by different techniques reporting low rate of minor complications but a complete lesion of the ulnar nerve. As Reddy described, we obtain the same low rate of complications using the technique previously presented,in a large series of patients (212 patients) operated by the same surgeon in 5 years (2004–2008) with an average follow up of 58 months with 1.8 % of neurological complications and 10.8 % of minor complications.

In 2001 Kelly et al. [17] reported extensive case studies in which they analysed complications following arthroscopic surgery. In some cases, other authors report limited case studies where they compare the outcomes achieved by open techniques with arthroscopic ones [20–28]. We believe that it is impossible to review any large series of elbow arthroscopies without report neurological complications, despite this we consider that 1.8 % of nervous complications can be defined as a low rate. We also think that 10.8 % of minor complications (sinovial leakage through the portals, superficial portal infections) are connected to our aggressive rehabilitative protocol. We still use this protocol because allows us to obtain a better ROM and results. In case of articular congruence damage, post-traumatic anatomical alterations or previous surgical outcome, arthroscopic indication is not common, while open surgery can be useful and decisive. On the other hand, arthroscopy is used in case of hypertrophy of the olecranon caused by long standing instability, radial head ostheophytes connected to a previous fracture, hypertrophy of the coronoid caused by an intense physical or manual activity. The use of 5 portals (3 posterior and 2 anterior) allows a clear and complete joint view. In our opinion, a complete view of anterior and posterior compartments is mandatory in any case, even if the pathology involves only one of the compartments. Even if the joint limitation affects only one of the two compartments, the lack of range of motion can lead to anatomo-pathological changes also in the other compartment, in the long run. As a result, there are many cases in which a radial head common compound fracture can cause joint stiffness due to posterior osteophytes and an increased radial head diameter. The use of retractors is important in every stage of the surgery because it minimizes any risk of damage to vascular and nervous structures. Intraarticular pressure should be always maintained below 50 mmHg by an arthroscopic pump. The number of portals allows the leakage of infused fluid, thus avoiding an excessive increase of intra-articular pressure within the joint. For this reason, the use of arthroscopic cannulas to keep all portals sealed (with the exception of the antero-lateral access) is contraindicated. During posterior debridement, the medial olecranon osteophytes removal should be carefully considered: a retractor can help, but in some cases due to big osteophytes proximity to the ulnar nerve, arthoscopic surgery is not recommended. The previous isolation of the ulnar nerve enables open surgery, avoiding risks. Posterior debridement and olecranon osteophytes removal allow an extension improvement that, together with the surgical procedures above mentioned, increases total ROM. Also anterior capsulectomy allows an extension improvement. On the contrary, flexion is favoured by posterior capsulectomy and removal of anterior hypertrophic coronoid or humeral osteophytes. During anterior capsulectomy, it is important to pay attention to the brachialis muscle which is visible once the capsule is removed and can be very thin as consequence of the stiffness. This is necessary not only because of the proximity of the humeral artery but also to avoid muscle bleeding, which can lead to possible calcifications. Taking into account the outcomes of a large series of patients we can assert that the ulnar nerve associated treatment has always been studied carefully. So far neurolysis has been performed in case of stiffness, with or without neurological disorders.

Only when ROM is almost complete and neurological disorders nearly absent, neurolisis is not performed (removal of 1–2 loose bodies). Anteposition of the ulnar nerve has never been carried out, except for one case in which the residual scar made it necessary. Once isolated, the nerve can be fixed anteriorly in cases of major stiffness, in severe valgus elbow or where a previous surgery prevents the proper positioning in the epitrocleo-olecranon fossa. Neurolysis of the ulnar nerve is nearly always recommended in cases of severe stiffness, and where there is a marked ROM recovery.

5.8   Results

The results reported in literature are extremely encouraging [10, 18, 20, 21, 25] allowing an increase ROM in both degenerative and post-traumatic cases. We obtained a quite satisfactory improved MEPI concerning the post-operative average 58 months follow up.

The average ROM improvement in post-traumatic forms was 35°, while in degenerative forms 33°. We have to remember that preoperative ROM in post-traumatic forms is lower than in degenerative forms. The improvement achieved allowed in 70.9 % of degenerative cases a total functional arc of movement higher than 100°.

Post-operative functional rehabilitation should be immediate to keep the intraoperative obtained ROM, thus reducing the inevitable risk of adhesions formation that can significantly limit the movement recovery. The suggested rehabilitation protocol can obviously be modified relatively to patient's needs in terms of more or less rehabilitation activity.

MEPI post-operative improvement was significantly showing a full recovery of working life, sports and relationships for the majority of patients. It also played a crucial role in the reduction of pain, as confirmed by both neurological evaluation and average VAS parameters. A comparable percentage improvement was observed in ROM recovery between post-traumatic and degenerative stiffness and those starting with a less severe Joint limitation.

As for ROM recovery, improvement was more considerable in extension than in flexion. This is due to the fact that anterior capsulectomy, the olecranon remodelling and the loose bodies removal lead to a higher increase of extension comparing to the coronoid osteophytes resection and the coronoid fossa trimming, which have mainly effects on elbow flexion.

Certainly, flexion may be limited by medial collateral ligament contractures. In this case we prefer to lyse the ligament in its posterior part through the open incision made for the ulnar neurolysis.

From the complications analysis, it is clear how common the presence of synovial fistulas is. These are related to the intense flexion–extension mobilization, which causes a synovial fluid leakage throughout surgical portals (locus minoris resistentiae), and prevents healing. In all cases, fistulas closed spontaneously 20 days after surgery [30]. During arthroscopy, the precaution of isolating the ulnar nerve before arthroscope introduction turned out to be extremely useful if compared to adverse outcomes when it was not performed. Retractors in the anterior compartment should not be used to detach the capsule but simply to remove the capsule itself and give the operator greater safety. If too much strength is used with the retractor, it can lead to excessive traction on the nerve structures.

5.9   Conclusions

Taking in consideration the high rate of success and low rate of complications in literature and in our personal experience we consider, in respect of literature indications, elbow arthroscopy as first choice treatment in stiff post-traumatic and degenerative elbows.

References

1. Andrews JR, Carson WG (1985) Arthroscopy of the elbow. Arthroscopy 1(2):97–107
2. Hempfling H (1983) Endoscopic examination of the elbow joint from the dorsoradial approach. Z Orthop Ihre Grenzgeb 121(3):331–332
3. Lindenfeld TN (1990) Medial approach in elbow arthroscopy. Am J Sports Med 18(4):413–417
4. Morrey BF, Askew LJ, Chao EY (1981) A biomechanical study of normal functional elbow motion. J Bone Joint Surg Am 63(6):872–877
5. O'Driscoll SW, Morrey BF (1992) Arthroscopy of the elbow. Diagnostic and therapeutic benefits and hazards. J Bone Joint Surg Am 74(1):84–94
6. Kelly EW, Morrey BF, O'Driscoll SW (2001) Complications of elbow arthroscopy. J Bone Joint Surg Am 83-A(1):25–34
7. Reddy AS, Kvitne RS, Yocum LA, ElAttrache NS, Glousman RE, Jobe FW (2000) Arthroscopy of the elbow: a long-term clinical review. Arthroscopy 16(6):588–594
8. Eames MHA, Bain GI (2006) Distal biceps tendon endoscopy and anterior elbow arthroscopy portal. Tech Shoulder Elbow Surg 7:139–142
9. Nirschl RP, Pettrone FA (1679) Tennis elbow: the surgical treatment of lateral epicondylitis. J Bone Joint Surg Am 61:832–839
10. Rahusen FT, Brinkman JM, Eygendaal D (2006) Results of arthroscopic debridement for osteochondritis dissecans of the elbow. Br J Sports Med 40(12):966–969
11. Savoie FH III (2007) Guidelines to becoming an expert elbow arthroscopist. Arthroscopy 23(11):1237–1240
12. Steinmann SP, King GJ, Savoie FH III (2006) Arthroscopic treatment of the arthritic elbow. Instr Course Lect 55:109–117
13. Akeson WH, Abel MF, Garfin SR, Woo SL (1993) Viscoelastic properties of stiff joints: a new approach in analyzing joint contracture. Biomed Mater Eng 3:67–73
14. Bruno RJ, Lee ML, Strauch RJ, Rosenwasser MP (2002) Posttraumatic elbow stiffness: evaluation and management. J Am Acad Orthop Surg 10(2):106–116

15. Morrey BF (2005) The posttraumatic stiff elbow. Clin Orthop Relat Res 431:26–35
16. Sojdjerg JO (1996) The stiff elbow. Acta Orthop Scand 67(6):626–631
17. Conso C, Bleton R (2007) Arthroscopy in stiff elbow: report of 32 cases. Rev Chir Orthop Reparatrice Appar Mot 93(4):333–338
18. Schubert T, Dubuc JE, Barbier O (2007) A review of 24 cases of elbow arthroscopy using the DASH questionnaire. Acta Orthop Belg 73(6):700–703
19. Salini V, Palmieri D, Colucci C, Croce G, Castellani ML, Orso CA (2006) Arthroscopic treatment of post-traumatic elbow stiffness. J Sports Med Phys Fitness 46(1):99–103
20. Adams JE, Wolff LH 3rd, Merten SM, Steinmann SP (2008) Osteoarthritis of the elbow: results of arthroscopic osteophyte resection and capsulectomy. J Shoulder Elbow Surg 17(1):126–131
21. Ball CM, Meunier M, Galatz LM, Calfee R, Yamaguchi K (2002) Arthroscopic treatment of post-traumatic elbow contracture. J Shoulder Elbow Surg 11(6):624–629
22. Figgie MP, Inglis AE, Mow CS, Figgie HE (1989) Total elbow arthroplasty for complete ankylosis of the elbow. J Bone Joint Surg Am 71:513–519
23. Guhl JF (1985) Arthroscopy and arthroscopic surgery of the elbow. Orthopedics 8:1290–1296
24. Lynch GJ, Meyers JF, Whipple TL, Caspari RB (1986) Neurovascular anatomy and elbow arthroscopy: inherent risks. Arthroscopy 2:190–197
25. Nguyen D, Proper SI, MacDermid JC, King GJ, Faber KJ (2006) Functional outcomes of arthroscopic capsular release of the elbow. Arthroscopy 22(8):842–849
26. Ogilvie-Harris DJ, Schemitsch E (1993) Arthroscopy of the elbow for removal of loose bodies. Arthroscopy 9:5–8
27. Rupp S, Tempelhof S (1995) Arthroscopic surgery of the elbow: therapeutic benefits and hazards. Clin Orthop 4:140–145
28. Ward WG, Anderson TE (1993) Elbow arthroscopy in a mostly athletic population. J Hand Surg Am 18:220–224
29. Savoie FH III (1996) Complication. In: Savoie FH III, Field LD (eds) Arthroscopy of the elbow. Churchill-Livingstone, New York, pp 151–156
30. Mader K, Penning D, Gausepohl T, Wulke AP (2004) Arthrolysis of the elbow joint. Unfallchirurg 107(5):403–411

The Role of Arthroscopy in Elbow Instability

6

Christian N. Anderson and Marc R. Safran

6.1 Valgus Elbow Instability

Valgus instability is a painful disorder of the medial elbow caused by acute or chronic ulnar collateral ligament (UCL) injury or attenuation. Injury to the UCL was first described by Waris [1] in a series of javelin throwers and since that time, has received increasing attention because of its disabling effects on athletes. Management of these injuries typically consists of a trial of non-operative treatment, and if unsuccessful, operative reconstruction can be considered. Although surgical reconstruction of the UCL is an open procedure, arthroscopy is useful in the diagnosis of valgus elbow instability and in the management of secondary conditions (valgus extension overload, loose bodies, and osteochondritis dissecans (OCD) of the capitellum) that arise as a result of chronic instability.

6.1.1 Anatomy and Pathophysiology

The UCL is a complex formed from three distinct bundles: the anterior oblique ligament (AOL), posterior oblique ligament (POL), and transverse ligament (Fig. 6.1) [2]. The AOL originates on the anterior inferior aspect of the medial epicondyle and inserts onto the sublime tubercle of the ulna [3]. The AOL has two histological layers—a deep layer within the medial capsule and a superficial layer on the surface of the capsule—and two functional bundles—the anterior and posterior bands [4]. The POL is a fan shaped capsular thickening that originates posterior to the AOL on the medial epicondyle and has a broad insertion on the

C. N. Anderson · M. R. Safran (✉)
Stanford University, 450 Broadway St., M/C 6342, Redwood City,
CA 94063, USA
e-mail: msafran@stanford.edu

L. A. Pederzini (ed.), *Elbow Arthroscopy*,
DOI: 10.1007/978-3-642-38103-4_6, © ISAKOS 2013

Fig. 6.1 Ulnar collateral ligament complex of the elbow (Reprinted with permission from Safran [40])

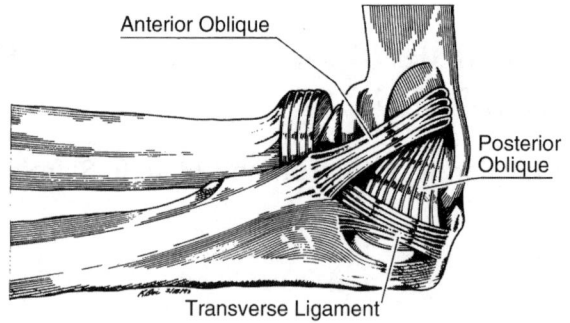

Anterior Oblique

Posterior Oblique

Transverse Ligament

medial edge of the olecranon [2]. The transverse ligament has a variable presence and spans the insertion of the AOL and POL on the medial ulna [5].

Valgus stability of the elbow is achieved through a complex interaction of dynamic and static soft tissue restraints and bony architecture. The primary anatomic structure providing valgus stability varies according to the degree of flexion at the elbow [6]. The AOL is the strongest component of the UCL [7] and provides the primary restraint to valgus stress during the throwing arc, between 20° and 120° of elbow flexion [8, 9]. The valgus stress at the elbow experienced during throwing and overhead sports produces significant forces on the UCL that approaches the ultimate tensile strength of the ligament [6, 10, 11]. These extreme forces coupled with the repetitive nature of overhead sports can result in microtrauma, ligament attenuation, and partial or complete rupture of the UCL.

Insufficiency of the UCL results in kinematic alterations that increase contact forces between the olecranon and posteromedial trochlea [12], leading a condition known as valgus extension overload [13]. In this condition, olecranon osteophytes and loose bodies form as a result of repetitive overloading of the posteromedial olecranon against the medial olecranon fossa wall, resulting in posteromedial elbow pain and decreased elbow extension as osteophytes enlarge (Fig. 6.2) [13, 14]. Incompetence of the UCL can also cause pathologic overloading of the radiocapitellar joint [11], as the radiocarpal joint is a secondary restraint to valgus forces [15]. This radiocapitellar compression may result in articular cartilage degeneration, osteophyte formation, osteochondral fracture, OCD of the capitellum, and loose body formation (Fig. 6.2).

6.1.2 History and Physical Exam

Injury to the UCL can be classified as acute, chronic, or acute on chronic. Athletes with an acute injury report a sudden onset of pain, often accompanied by a "pop" at the medial elbow, during overhead activity that prevents return to play. Chronic valgus instability is caused by gradual ligamentous attenuation and manifests as medial elbow pain, decreased stamina and strength, and loss of ball control and velocity during overhead activity. Athletes may have symptoms of ulnar

Fig. 6.2 Posteriorly, the olecranon is subjected to medial shearing forces with valgus stress, which may be accentuated by increased valgus laxity, resulting in valgus extension overload with osteophyte formation and loose bodies (Reprinted with permission from Safran [41])

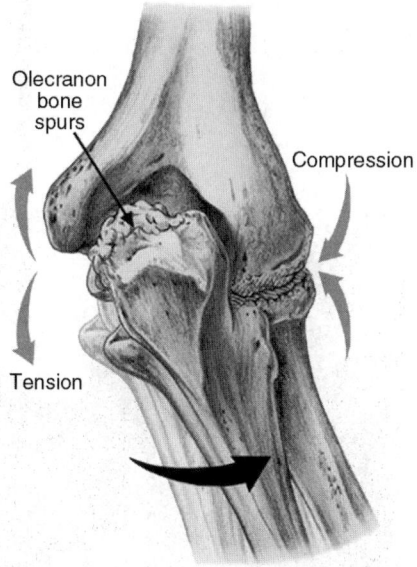

neuropathy from either acute or chronic UCL injury caused by edema/hemorrhage of the medial elbow or excessive traction on the nerve. Valgus extension overload and resulting loose bodies can cause symptoms of catching or locking at the elbow, and manipulation may be needed to release or unlock it.

The physical exam begins with a general inspection, palpation, and active and passive range-of-motion of the upper extremity joints. Patients with isolated UCL injury often have point tenderness 2 cm distal to the medial epicondyle, slightly posterior to the common flexor origin. A thorough neurovascular exam of the upper extremity should be obtained to rule out ulnar neuropathy.

The integrity of the UCL can be assessed with specific physical exam tests. The "milking maneuver" involves having the patient apply a valgus torque to the elbow by pulling down on the thumb of the injured extremity with the contralateral limb providing stability (Fig. 6.3) [16]. With the modified milking maneuver, the examiner provides stability to the patient's elbow and pulls the thumb to create a valgus stress on the UCL (Fig. 6.4) [17]. These tests result in pain and widening at the medial joint line if the UCL is insufficient. O'Driscoll and coworkers described the moving valgus stress test, whereby the examiner applies and maintains a constant valgus torque to the fully flexed elbow, then quickly extends the elbow [18]. This test is positive if medial elbow pain is elicited and has a 100 % sensitivity and 75 % specificity [18]. The abduction valgus stress test is performed by stabilizing the patient's abducted and externally rotated arm with the examiners axilla and applying a valgus force to the elbow at 30° of flexion (Fig. 6.5). Testing with the forearm in neutral rotation has been show to elicit the greatest valgus instability [19]. A positive test results in medial elbow pain and widening along the medial joint line. Even so, valgus laxity can be subtle on physical exam and the range of preoperative detection

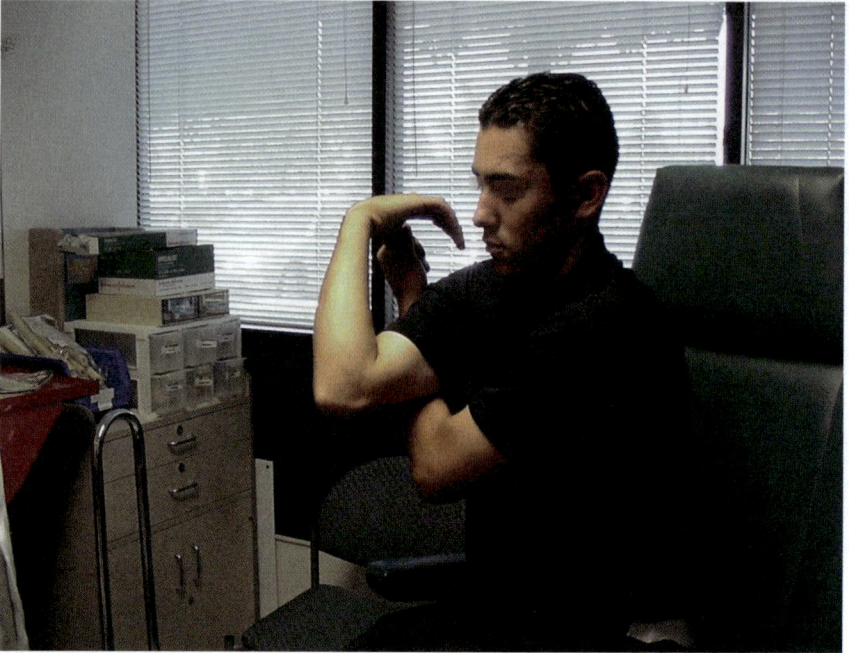

Fig. 6.3 The "milking maneuver." The patient's contralateral arm stabilizes the shoulder of the injured extremity and applies a valgus torque to the elbow by pulling on the thumb of the extremity being examined. The examiner then palpates the medial joint line for gapping (Reprinted with permission from Hariri [42])

is between 26 and 82 % of patients [20, 21]. Furthermore, Timmerman and colleagues found valgus stress testing to be only 66 % sensitive and 60 % specific for detecting abnormality of the anterior bundle of the UCL [22].

6.1.3 Arthroscopic Diagnosis

Arthroscopy has emerged as an important tool to confirm the diagnosis of valgus instability of the elbow. Unfortunately, only portions of the UCL itself can be visualized during arthroscopy. In a cadaveric study, Timmerman and Andrews demonstrated that only 20–30 % of the AOL was visible through the anterolateral portal and 30–50 % of the POL could be visualized via the posterolateral portal (Fig. 6.6) [4]. Viewing from the anterolateral portal, with the elbow at 70° they found the ulnohumeral joint opens less than 1 mm to valgus stress with an intact AOL. Complete sectioning of the AOL resulted in a 3–5 mm opening of the ulnohumeral joint with a valgus stress (Fig. 6.7). Field and Altcheck also arthroscopically quantified medial gapping relative to UCL sectioning in cadavers and found no opening for intact AOL and 1–2 mm of widening after transecting the AOL [23]. These studies suggest that while a direct arthroscopic assessment of the

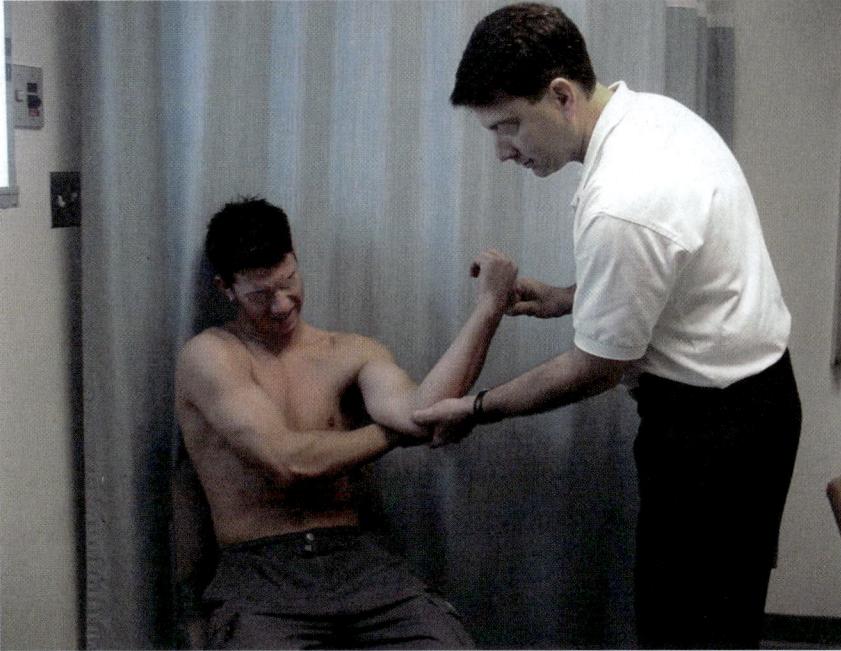

Fig. 6.4 The senior author's modification of the milking maneuver. The patient still locks the shoulder of the upper extremity being examined by using the other arm. The examiner positions the patient's elbow at 70° and pulls on the subject's thumb to impart the valgus stress while palpating the medial joint line with the other hand (Reprinted with permission from Hariri [42])

status of the AOL is difficult, arthroscopy can be used to indirectly determine AOL insufficiency by quantifying medial ulnohumeral joint opening with valgus stress. After the diagnosis of AOL insufficiency is confirmed arthroscopically, open reconstruction can be performed to stabilize the medial elbow.

6.1.4   Arthroscopic Treatment

The complex bony geometry of the elbow coupled with the extra-articular insertional anatomy of the UCL and close proximity of the ulnar nerve precludes arthroscopic reconstruction of the AOL. Even so, arthroscopy can be used as an important tool in treating the long-term sequelae of UCL insufficiency. Posteromedial olecranon osteophytes that result from valgus extension overload can be removed arthroscopically with less morbidity than open arthrotomy.

It is important to note that patients with valgus extension overload should be thoroughly evaluated for UCL insufficiency. Andrews and Timmerman reported 25 % of baseball players developed instability and required UCL reconstruction after olecranon debridement [24]. It is unclear if these patients had preexisting

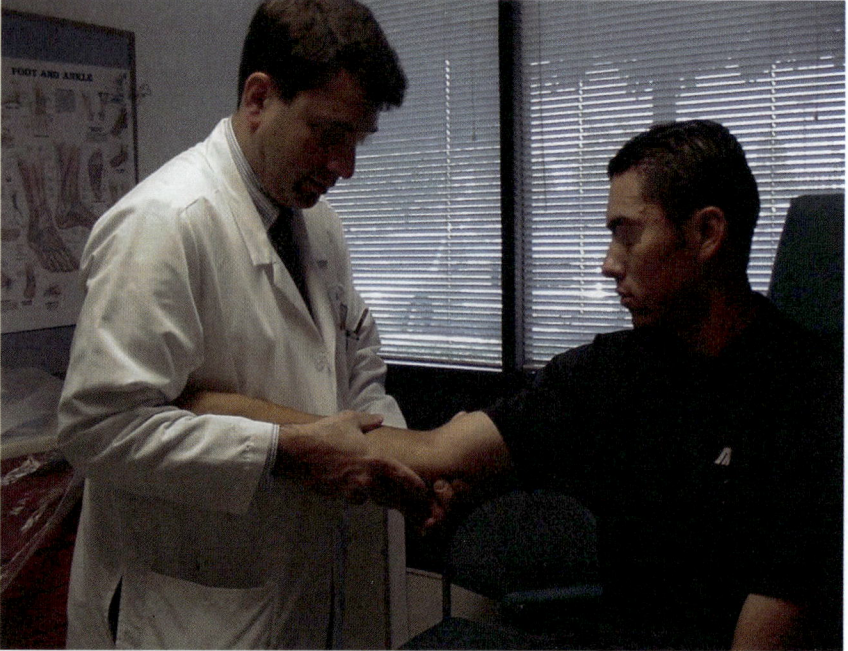

Fig. 6.5 Abduction valgus stress test. A valgus stress is applied to the elbow flexed 30°, palpating the UCL for tenderness and opening of the medial joint line (Reprinted with permission from Hariri [42])

Fig. 6.6 Portions of the anterior and posterior oblique ligaments that can be visualized arthroscopically (Reprinted with permission from Timmerman and Andrews [4])

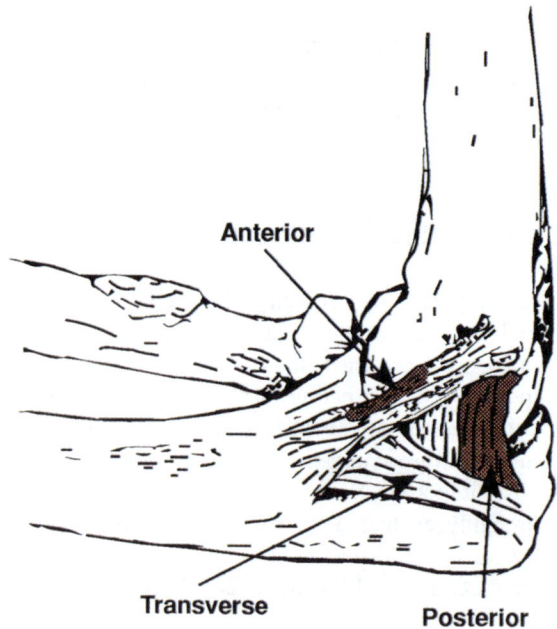

Anterior

Transverse

Posterior

Fig. 6.7 Ulnohumeral joint widening with valgus stress to the elbow (Courtesy of Marc Safran, MD, Redwood City, CA.)

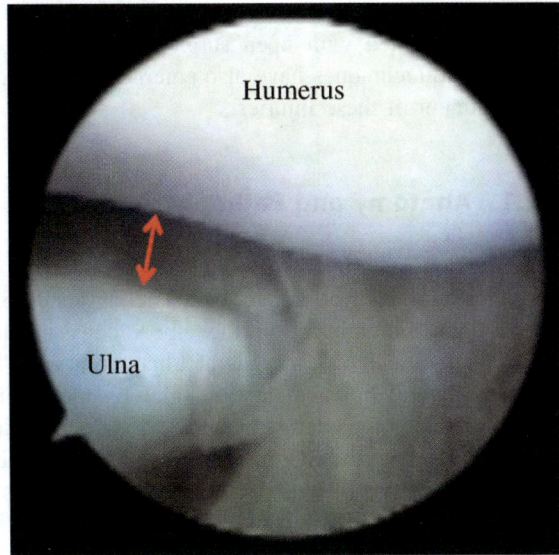

valgus instability that manifested after removal of stabilizing osteophytes or if removal of the osteophytes caused additional ligamentous overload. Nevertheless, biomechanical studies have demonstrated a stepwise increase in UCL strain and valgus instability with sequential partial resection of the posteromedial olecranon [25, 26]. These studies suggest posterior debridement should be limited to removal of osteophytes only to preserve the stabilizing function of the ulna.

Loose bodies may also be removed more easily and with less morbidity arthroscopically as compared with open loose body removal. CT Arthrography and/or MRI may help in identifying the number and location of the loose bodies, however they may move by the time surgery is undertaken. The number of loose bodies identified on imaging studies can be helpful, as the surgeon should remove at least the number identified on these pre-operative studies, though more, smaller ones may exist. Anterior loose bodies are usually found around the proximal radioulnar joint, while posterior loose bodies can be found in the posteromedial and posterolateral gutters, as well as the olecranon fossa.

6.2   Posterolateral Rotatory Instability

Posterolateral rotatory instability is a clinical syndrome of the elbow first described in 1991 by O'Driscoll and colleagues in a series of five patients [27]. PLRI is most commonly caused by a traumatic injury to the lateral collateral ligament (LCL) complex after acute elbow subluxation or dislocation and results in recurrent lateral elbow pain and instability. Treatment after acute elbow dislocation typically consists wearing a hinged elbow brace for 4–6 weeks with the forearm in full pronation. Patients that develop recurrent instability after nonsurgical management have been treated with open surgical reconstruction or repair. More recently, arthroscopic techniques have also emerged as an important tool for the diagnosis and treatment of these injuries.

6.2.1 Anatomy and Pathophysiology

Lateral elbow stability is maintained by an interaction of static and dynamic soft tissue restraints as well as the osseous congruency of the elbow. The lateral collateral ligament complex of the elbow consists of four structures—the radial collateral ligament (RCL), lateral ulnar collateral ligament (LUCL), accessory lateral collateral ligament, and annular ligament (Fig. 6.8) [2]. The LUCL and RCL originate at the lateral epicondyle and are indistinct at that location. From the lateral epicondyle, the RCL extends distally and blends with the annular ligament, which inserts along the anterior and posterior margins of the radial notch [28]. The LUCL extends distally to insert directly onto a tubercle of the supinator crest—the crista supinatoris [2].

Controlled laboratory studies have been conducted to determine the relative contributions the lateral structures have on elbow stability. McAdams and coworkers sectioned the RCL and LUCL arthroscopically in cadaveric specimens and found no instability with sectioning ligaments independently; however, when both ligaments were released instability was noted with pivot shift testing [29]. Furthermore, they found releasing the common extensor origin after release of the ulnar collateral ligaments further destabilized the elbow, resulting in complete instability [29]. Cohen and Hastings determined the lateral collateral ligament complex was the primary restraint to PLRI and secondary restraint was provided by extensor muscles, fascial bands, and the intermuscular septum [28]. Dunning and colleagues also demonstrated that sectioning of both the RCL and LUCL was

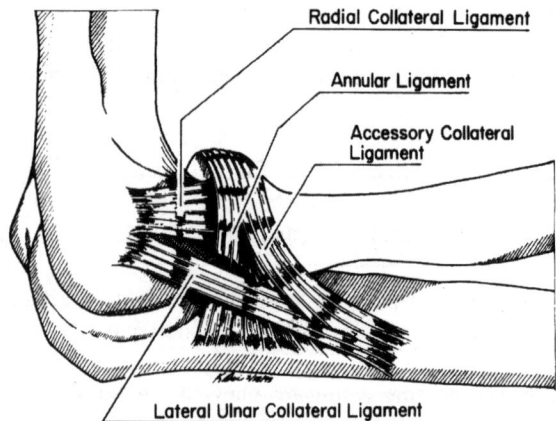

Fig. 6.8 Anatomy of the lateral ligaments of the elbow (Reprinted with permission from Safran [40])

necessary to induce elbow instability [30]. While differences exist between cadaveric models and in clinical scenarios, two thirds of patients requiring surgery for PLRI have both ligamentous and extensor tendon disruption from the lateral epicondyle, providing further evidence of the importance of both muscular and ligamentous structures in lateral elbow stability [31].

The clinical mechanism of injury to the lateral stabilizers of the elbow that results in PLRI has been hypothesized to consist of supination the forearm, combined with a valgus and axial load to the elbow [32]. This combination of forces results in circumferential disruption of the ligaments and capsule around the elbow joint. In stage I, the LCL complex is disrupted, resulting in PLRI manifested by radiocapitellar and ulnohumeral joint subluxation. In stage II, the forces are transmitted to the remaining intact structures—the anterior and posterior joint capsules—resulting in capsular disruption and an incomplete "perched" dislocation. In stage III, the POL of the medial ulnar collateral ligament is disrupted, leaving the AOL intact, resulting in posterior elbow dislocation.

6.2.2   History and Physical Exam

Patients with PLRI most commonly have a history of previous elbow dislocation or trauma; however, PLRI has also been reported with chronic cubitus varus deformity [33] and after aggressive release for lateral epicondylitis [34]. The presentation is variable and can include lateral elbow pain, mechanical symptoms such as snapping, clicking, catching or locking, and recurrent episodes of instability. Patients often report their elbow feels loose or like it is sliding out of place, especially when loading it in a slightly flexed position with a supinated forearm, as when pushing off an armrest while standing from a chair.

On physical exam, patients often have normal upper extremity strength and elbow range of motion, and minimal to no tenderness around the LCL complex. While PLRI can be difficult to detect on routine physical examination, several provocative maneuvers have been developed to elicit instability symptoms. The posterolateral rotatory instability test is performed by supinating the forearm and applying valgus and axial forces to the elbow, while flexing the elbow from full extension (Fig. 6.9) [27]. A positive test is demonstrated by reduction of a subluxed radial head when the patient is under general anesthesia or apprehension during testing when the patient is awake [27]. More recently, Regan and Lapner described two other apprehension tests, the chair sign and push-up sign [35]. The chair sign is performed by having the patient actively push off armrests of a chair with the forearms supinated and the elbows at 90° (Fig. 6.10). The test is considered positive with reluctance to fully extend the elbow during push off. The push-up sign is conducted by having the patient push off from the ground with the forearms supinated, elbows at 90°, and arms abducted to greater than shoulder width (Fig. 6.11). A positive test results in apprehension and guarding as the elbow is terminally extended. These apprehension tests have been determined to be more sensitive than the posterolateral rotator instability test in awake patients [35].

6.2.3 Arthroscopic Diagnosis

Arthroscopy is a useful tool for the diagnosis of suspected cases of PLRI where physical exam is not conclusive. After routine diagnostic arthroscopy, the radio-capitellar joint is viewed from the anteromedial portal, while simultaneously supinating the forearm with the elbow flexed 90° [36]. Patients with PLRI will have rotation and posterior subluxation of the radial head on the capitellum with testing, while normal patients will have rotation without subluxation (Fig. 6.12) [36]. This can also be seen when performing arthroscopy from the posterior compartment. With the arthroscope in the posterolateral gutter, the forearm can be supinated with the elbow flexed, demonstrating the subluxation of the radial head posteriorly. Patients with PLRI will also have a positive "drive-through sign", whereby the arthroscope can be driven through the lateral gutter from the posterolateral portal into the lateral aspect of the ulnohumeral joint [37].

6.2.4 Arthroscopic Treatment

For patients refractory to non-operative treatment that develop functional impairment from PLRI, arthroscopic LCL complex repair and plication techniques have been developed [36, 38, 39]. Arthroscopic repair can be performed for patients with acute or chronic avulsion of the LCL complex from its humeral origin [38]. Viewing from the posterocentral portal, the site of ligament avulsion is localized on the lateral aspect of the posterior humerus, usually directly lateral and slightly inferior to the olecranon fossa. A suture anchor is then placed in the humerus at the origin of the native LCL complex. Sutures are then passed through the non-injured portion of the ligament and tied under the anconeus muscle with the elbow in full extension, thereby repairing the native ligament to its humeral origin.

Arthroscopic plication is usually performed for chronic attenuation of the LCL complex [36, 38, 39]. This technique is performed by placing four to seven absorbable sutures in an obliquely oriented fashion through the LCL complex, starting distally where the ligament attaches to the ulna and moving progressively proximal with subsequent sutures. Suture tag ends are passed underneath the LCL complex origin on the humerus and tied outside the capsule through a small skin incision sequentially to tension the ligament. If the patient continues to have posterior subluxation with posterolateral rotatory instability testing after plication, a suture anchor can be placed at the isometric point of the lateral epicondyle and used to pull the entire plicated complex back to the humeral origin. Savoie and

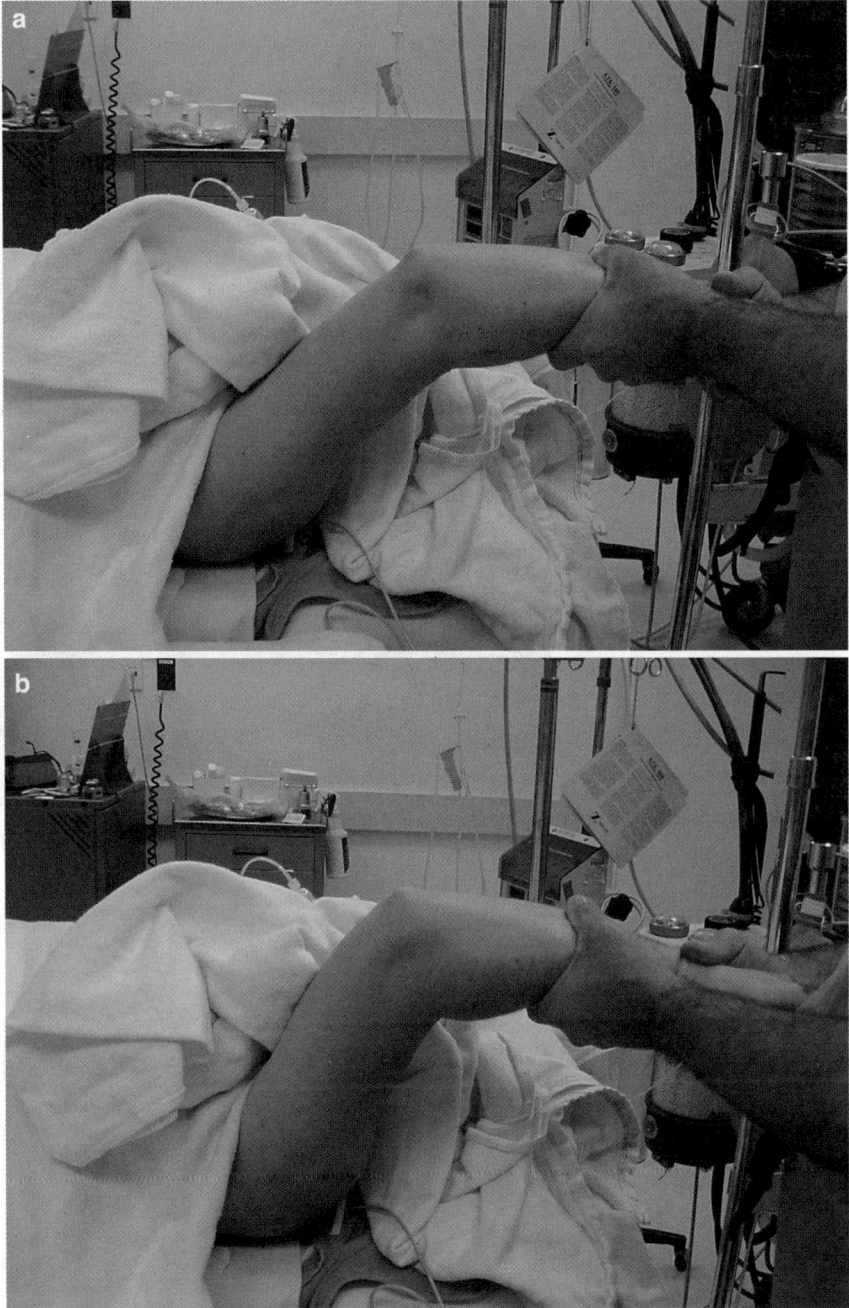

Fig. 6.9 The posterolateral rotatory instability test. The forearm is supinated and a valgus and axial load is applied to the extended elbow (**a**). The elbow is then flexed (**b**) and the radial head is reduced if PLRI is present (Courtesy of Marc Safran, MD, Redwood City, CA.)

Fig. 6.10 The chair sign.
The patient actively pushes
off armrests of a chair with
the forearms supinated and
the elbows at 90° (**a**). The test
is positive with reluctance to
fully extend the elbow
(**b**) (Courtesy of Marc Safran,
MD, Redwood City, CA.)

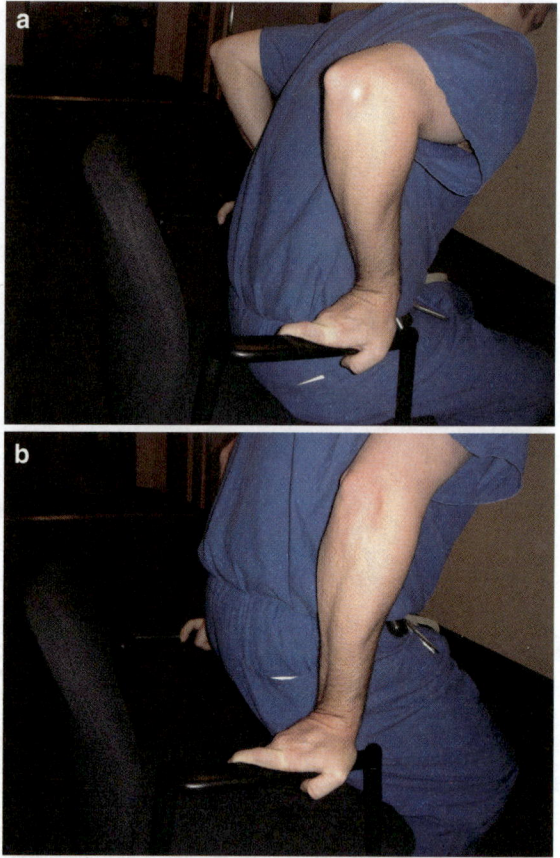

Fig. 6.11 The push-up sign.
The patient performs a push-
up with hands supinated. A
positive test is noted by
apprehension with elbow
extension (Courtesy of Marc
Safran, MD, Redwood City,
CA.)

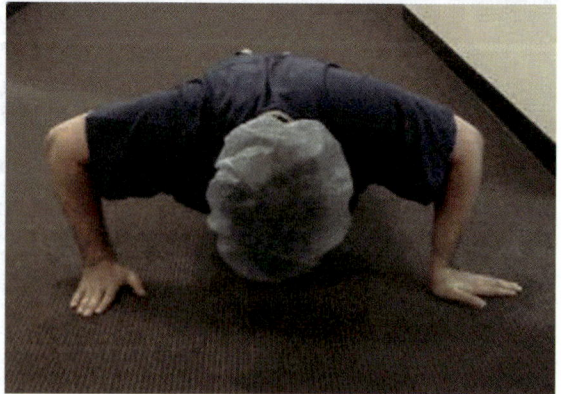

Fig. 6.12 Posterior subluxation of the radial head seen arthroscopically from the posterior portal while performing the posterolateral rotatory instability test (Courtesy of Marc Safran, MD, Redwood City, CA.)

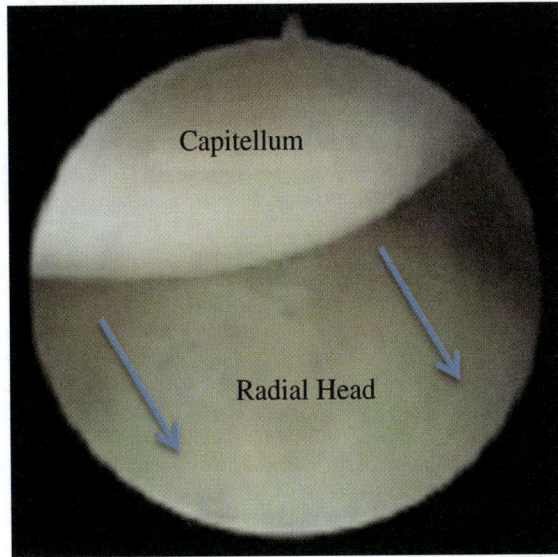

colleagues reported on 61 patients undergoing surgery for PLRI and found both arthroscopic and open techniques significantly improved subjective and objective outcomes [38].

References

1. Waris W (1946) Elbow injuries of javelin-throwers. Acta chirurgica Scandinavica 93:563–575
2. Morrey BF, An KN (1985) Functional anatomy of the ligaments of the elbow. Clin Orthop 201:84–90
3. O'Driscoll SW, Jaloszynski R, Morrey BF et al (1992) Origin of the medial ulnar collateral ligament. J Hand Surg [Am] 17:164–168
4. Timmerman LA, Andrews JR (1994) Histology and arthroscopic anatomy of the ulnar collateral ligament of the elbow. Am J Sports Med 22:667–673
5. Fuss FK (1991) The ulnar collateral ligament of the human elbow joint. Anatomy, function and biomechanics. J Anat 175:203–212
6. Morrey BF, An KN (1983) Articular and ligamentous contributions to the stability of the elbow joint. Am J Sports Med 11:315–319
7. Regan WD, Korinek SL, Morrey BF et al (1991) Biomechanical study of ligaments around the elbow joint. Clin Orthop 271:170–179
8. Callaway GH, Field LD, Deng XH et al (1997) Biomechanical evaluation of the medial collateral ligament of the elbow. J Bone Joint Surg Am 79:1223–1231
9. Morrey BF, Tanaka S, An KN (1991) Valgus stability of the elbow. A definition of primary and secondary constraints. Clin Orthop 265:187–195
10. Ahmad CS, Lee TQ, Elattrache NS (2003) Biomechanical evaluation of a new ulnar collateral ligament reconstruction technique with interference screw fixation. Am J Sports Med 31:332–337

11. Fleisig GS, Andrews JR, Dillman CJ et al (1995) Kinetics of baseball pitching with implications about injury mechanisms. Am J Sports Med 23:233–239
12. Ahmad CS (2004) Elbow medial ulnar collateral ligament insufficiency alters posteromedial olecranon contact. Am J Sports Med 32:1607–1612
13. Wilson FD, Andrews JR, Blackburn TA et al (1983) Valgus extension overload in the pitching elbow. Am J Sports Med 11:83–88
14. Rahusen FT, Brinkman JM, Eygendaal D (2009) Arthroscopic treatment of posterior impingement of the elbow in athletes: a medium-term follow-up in sixteen cases. J Shoulder Elbow Surg 18:279–282
15. Hotchkiss RN, Weiland AJ (1987) Valgus stability of the elbow. J Orthop Res 5:372–377
16. Safran MR (2004) Ulnar collateral ligament injury in the overhead athlete: diagnosis and treatment. Clin Sports Med 23:643–663
17. Safran MR, Caldwell GL, Fu FH (1996) Chronic instability of the elbow. In Peimer CA (ed) Surgery of the hand and upper extremity. McGraw-Hill, New York, pp 467–490
18. O'Driscoll SWM, Lawton RL, Smith AM (2005) the moving valgus stress test for medial collateral ligament tears of the elbow. Am J Sports Med 33:231–239
19. Safran MR, Mcgarry MH, Shin S et al (2005) Effects of elbow flexion and forearm rotation on valgus laxity of the elbow. J Bone Joint Surg Am 87:2065–2074
20. Azar FM, Andrews JR, Wilk KE et al (2000) Operative treatment of ulnar collateral ligament injuries of the elbow in athletes. Am J Sports Med 28:16–23
21. Thompson W (2001) Ulnar collateral ligament reconstruction in athletes: muscle-splitting approach without transposition of the ulnar nerve. J Shoulder Elbow Surg 10:152–157
22. Timmerman LA, Schwartz ML, Andrews JR (1994) Preoperative evaluation of the ulnar collateral ligament by magnetic resonance imaging and computed tomography arthrography. Evaluation in 25 baseball players with surgical confirmation. Am J Sports Med 32:26–31
23. Field LD, Altchek DW (1996) Evaluation of the arthroscopic valgus instability test of the elbow. Am J Sports Med 24:177–181
24. Andrews JR, Timmerman LA (1995) Outcome of elbow surgery in professional baseball players. Am J Sports Med 23:407–413
25. Kamineni S, Elattrache NS, O'Driscoll SW et al (2004) medial collateral ligament strain with partial posteromedial olecranon resection. A biomechanical study. J Bone Joint Surg Am 86:2424–2430
26. Kamineni S, Hirahara H, Pomianowski S et al (2003) Partial posteromedial olecranon resection: a kinematic study. J Bone Joint Surg Am 85:1005–1011
27. O'Driscoll SW, Bell DF, Morrey BF (1991) Posterolateral rotatory instability of the elbow. J Bone Joint Surg Am 73:440–446
28. Cohen MS, Hastings H (1997) Rotatory instability of the elbow. The anatomy and role of the lateral stabilizers. J Bone Joint Surg Am 79:225–233
29. Mcadams TR, Masters GW, Srivastava S (2005) The effect of arthroscopic sectioning of the lateral ligament complex of the elbow on posterolateral rotatory stability. J Shoulder Elbow Surg 14:298–301
30. Dunning CE, Zarzour ZD, Patterson SD et al (2001) Ligamentous stabilizers against posterolateral rotatory instability of the elbow. J Bone Joint Surg Am 83A:1823–1828
31. Mckee MD, Schemitsch EH, Sala MJ et al (2003) The pathoanatomy of lateral ligamentous disruption in complex elbow instability. J Shoulder Elbow Surg 12:391–396
32. O'Driscoll SW, Morrey BF, Korinek S et al (1992) Elbow subluxation and dislocation. A spectrum of instability. Clin Orthop. 280:186–197
33. O'Driscoll SW, Spinner RJ, Mckee MD et al (2001) Tardy posterolateral rotatory instability of the elbow due to cubitus varus. J Bone Joint Surg Am 83A:1358–1369
34. Morrey BF (1992) Reoperation for failed surgical treatment of refractory lateral epicondylitis. J Shoulder Elbow Surg 1:47–55
35. Regan W, Lapner PC (2006) Prospective evaluation of two diagnostic apprehension signs for posterolateral instability of the elbow. J Shoulder Elbow Surg 15:344–346

36. Smith JP, Savoie FH 3rd, Field LD (2001) Posterolateral rotatory instability of the elbow. Clin Sports Med 20:47–58
37. Yadao MA, Savoie FH 3rd, Field LD (2004) Posterolateral rotatory instability of the elbow. Instr Course Lect 53:607–614
38. Savoie FH 3rd, Field LD, Gurley DJ (2009) Arthroscopic and open radial ulnohumeral ligament reconstruction for posterolateral rotatory instability of the elbow. Hand Clin 25:323–329
39. Savoie FH 3rd, O'Brien MJ, Field LD, Gurley DJ (2010) Arthroscopic and open radial ulnohumeral ligament reconstruction for posterolateral rotatory instability of the elbow. Clin Sports Med 29:611–618
40. Safran MR (1995) Elbow injuries in athletes. Clin Orthop 310:260
41. Safran MR (2003) Injury to the ulnar collateral ligament: diagnosis and treatment. Sports Med Arthrosc Rev 11:17
42. Hariri S, Safran MS (2010) Ulnar collateral ligament injury in the overhead athlete. Clin Sports Med 29(4):619–644

Endoscopy Around the Elbow

7

Duncan Thomas McGuire and Gregory Ian Bain

7.1 Introduction

Arthroscopy of the elbow joint is well established. However, soft tissue endoscopy around the elbow is relatively new, having been made possible by new techniques and advances in equipment design. As techniques evolve and evidence supporting these techniques is published, soft tissue endoscopy around the elbow may become common practice.

Before any soft tissue endoscopic procedure is attempted familiarity with the open technique is essential. A "backup" is required for both patient safety and in the event that the arthroscopic procedure cannot be completed. The open techniques are also the gold standard by which other minimally invasive procedures will be measured. The greatest concern with these procedures is neurovascular damage due to the proximity of these structures. Thus, a thorough understanding of the surgical anatomy of the elbow is paramount.

Endoscopy may be performed wet or dry. Wet endoscopy is similar to arthroscopy in which resectors, burrs and cautery may be used. Fluid distension is used to enlarge the viewing cavity and to wash away the debris. Dry endoscopy avoids fluid extravasation, but relies on other methods of distension.

D. T. McGuire · G. I. Bain
Department of Orthopaedics and Trauma, Royal Adelaide Hospital, Adelaide, SA, Australia

G. I. Bain (✉)
Department of Orthopaedics and Trauma, University of Adelaide, Adelaide, SA, Australia
e-mail: greg@gregbain.com.au; gregbain@internode.on.net

L. A. Pederzini (ed.), *Elbow Arthroscopy*,
DOI: 10.1007/978-3-642-38103-4_7, © ISAKOS 2013

7.2   Endoscopic Cubital Tunnel Release

Ulnar nerve entrapment at the level of the elbow is the second most common entrapment neuropathy in the upper limb behind carpal tunnel syndrome [1, 2]. Treatment options include open and endoscopic cubital tunnel release with or without anterior transposition of the ulnar nerve. Meta-analyses have reported that in situ decompression has comparable outcomes with anterior transposition but with fewer complications [3, 4]. An endoscopic decompression has been shown to be as effective as the open decompression, however has the advantages of being less invasive, a smaller incision, less vascular insult to the nerve and faster recovery [1, 5]. A prospective study comparing the outcomes of the two techniques, reported better patient satisfaction with the endoscopic technique and a lower complication rate, including elbow pain, scar tenderness and medial elbow paraesthesia [1].

The common sites of ulnar nerve compression are the arcade of Struthers; the cubital tunnel (most common); and the FCU fascia which extends from an average of 8 cm proximal, and 5 cm distal, to the medial epicondyle [2]. The indication for endoscopic cubital tunnel release is failed conservative management of cubital tunnel syndrome. Contraindications to endoscopic release include: space-occupying lesions, previous ulnar nerve release or transposition, and severe elbow contractures requiring release [1, 6]. An unstable ulnar nerve requires an anterior transposition, which can now be performed as an endoscopic procedure.

Several endoscopic techniques for ulnar nerve release have been described. The authors' published the technique utilising the Agee Micro-Aire endoscopic carpal tunnel device [2]. This device has a pistol grip hand-piece with a trigger that activates a retractable cutting blade from a protected sheath immediately distal to the endoscopic tip. This allows direct visualisation of the blade and the tissue that is to be transected. The blade may be quickly and simply retracted out of harm's way by releasing the trigger mechanism. A cadaveric study has demonstrated the safety and reproducibility of this technique [2].

7.2.1   Surgical Technique: Endoscopic Cubital Tunnel Release

Under general anaesthesia, the patient is placed in the lateral decubitus position with the operative arm over a padded bolster and an upper arm tourniquet inflated. No irrigation is required as this is a dry endoscopic technique. A 3 cm longitudinal incision is made between the medial epicondyle and olecranon. Blunt dissection is performed to the level of the cubital retinaculum, the fibres of which run perpendicular to those of the aponeurosis of flexor carpi ulnaris. A small fenestration is made in the retinaculum and the Agee device is introduced into the cubital tunnel, adjacent to the nerve under direct vision (Fig. 7.1a). The device is then employed both proximally and distally to release all overlying constrictive tissues, ensuring that the retinaculum is visible at all times and the nerve and its branches

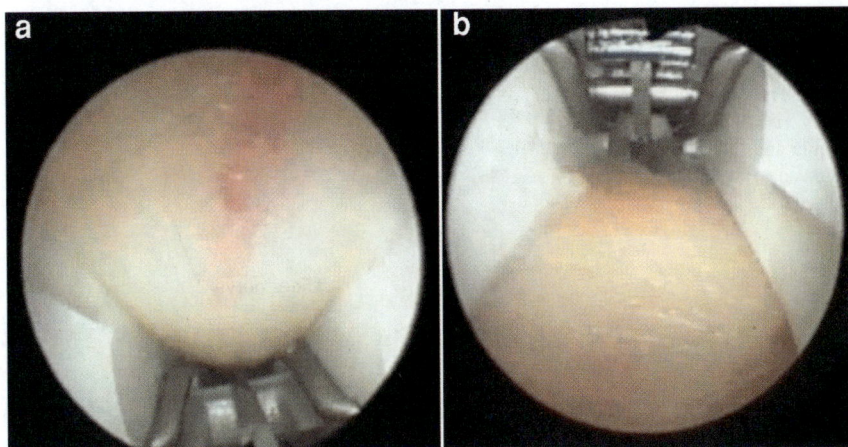

Fig. 7.1 **a** Endoscopic ulnar nerve release with Agee device, scope introduced with the ulnar nerve and its vessels on view through the aperture. **b** Endoscopic ulnar nerve release, the scope and cannula has been rotated to protect the nerve and to expose the retinaculum. The trigger is activated to engage the knife. Withdrawal of the device with the knife engaged will incise the cubital retinaculum

are not threatened [1, 2] (Fig. 7.1b). The device is then reintroduced to assess the adequacy of the decompression. Rehabilitation consists of early active range of motion activities and return to normal activities as tolerated.

Other techniques include those by Hoffman (Storz), Cobb (Integra) and Tsai (glass tubes) [6–8]. The Hoffman technique utilises a set of instruments originally developed for endoscopic facelift surgery [7]. A tunnelling forceps is used to open the subcutaneous plane, into which a hooded endoscope is introduced, which acts as a tent post, to keep open the working endoscopic space, into which scissors and cautery can be introduced. Cobb's technique utilises the Integra EndoRelease system that has a cannula specifically designed for cubital tunnel release. The ulnar nerve is protected under this cannula while the roof of the cubital tunnel is released [6]. Tsai utilised glass tubes to house an endoscope and guide a meniscus knife [8] (Fig. 7.2a and b).

7.2.2 Surgical Technique: Endoscopic Ulnar Nerve Transposition

The subcutaneous plane at the level of the deep fascia is elevated anterior to the medial epicondyle. The standard endoscopic ulnar nerve release is performed. The medial intermuscular septum is then identified and released. Care is taken to ensure that any adjacent vessels are protected or cauterised. The ulnar nerve is then mobilised and transferred anterior to the medial epicondyle. The incised deep fascia over the proximal forearm can be repaired with barbed sutures, to prevent herniation, which are inserted endoscopically and do not require ligation. The

Fig. 7.2 **a** and **b** Technique of endoscopic ulnar nerve release using the Integra device. The ulnar nerve is clearly visualized *below* the cannula and the blade advanced to divide the fascia *above*

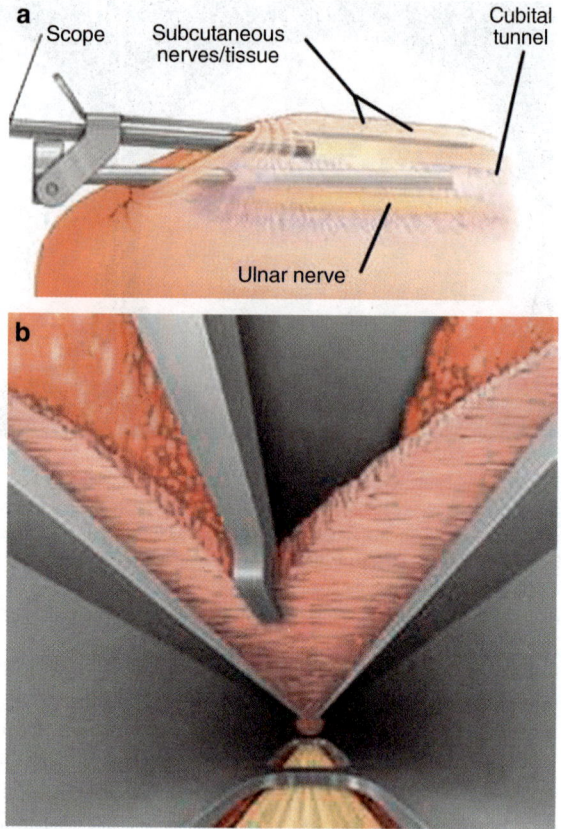

nerve should be checked proximally and distally to ensure that there is no kinking of the nerve. Once this is confirmed and an adequate bed has been prepared for the nerve, the subcutaneous fat is then sutured to the soft tissue over the medial epicondyle. The elbow is placed into a sling in flexion for one week to ensure that the soft tissues heal, and to stabilise the nerve in its new bed.

The authors have also performed releases of the proximal median nerve and radial nerve, where the initial exposure is open to identify the nerve, and then perform the remainder of the release as an endoscopic procedure. This reduces the morbidity of the procedure, while preserving its safety.

7.3   Olecranon Bursoscopy

Olecranon bursitis is the most common form of superficial bursitis at the elbow [9]. Septic bursitis accounts for a third and sterile bursitis about two-thirds of all cases [10]. The two conditions can be differentiated on clinical grounds. Septic olecranon bursitis is usually caused by Staphylococcus Aureus [11] and requires bacterial culture, drainage, irrigation and antibiotics. This can all be performed as a wet endoscopic procedure, with portals proximal and distal to the bursa, with the granulation tissue endoscopically resected and the portals left open to encourage drainage of any purulent fluid.

Sterile olecranon bursitis can result from local repetitive trauma, rheumatoid arthritis, gout, hydroxyapatite crystal disease and chondrocalcinosis [11, 12]. Surgery is indicated when conservative treatment fails, and traditionally involves an open excision of the bursa, but wound healing can really be a problem. The endoscopic technique can be performed as a wet or dry procedure, and utilises incisions away from the point of the olecranon preserving the bridging skin and heals more quickly than the open technique.

The wet endoscopic technique involves introducing the arthroscopic equipment into the bursa and resecting it from inside out, until normal tissue is left. Good results, including faster wound healing, lower re-operation rate and a shorter hospital stay have been reported with this technique [13, 14] (Fig. 7.3a). The dry

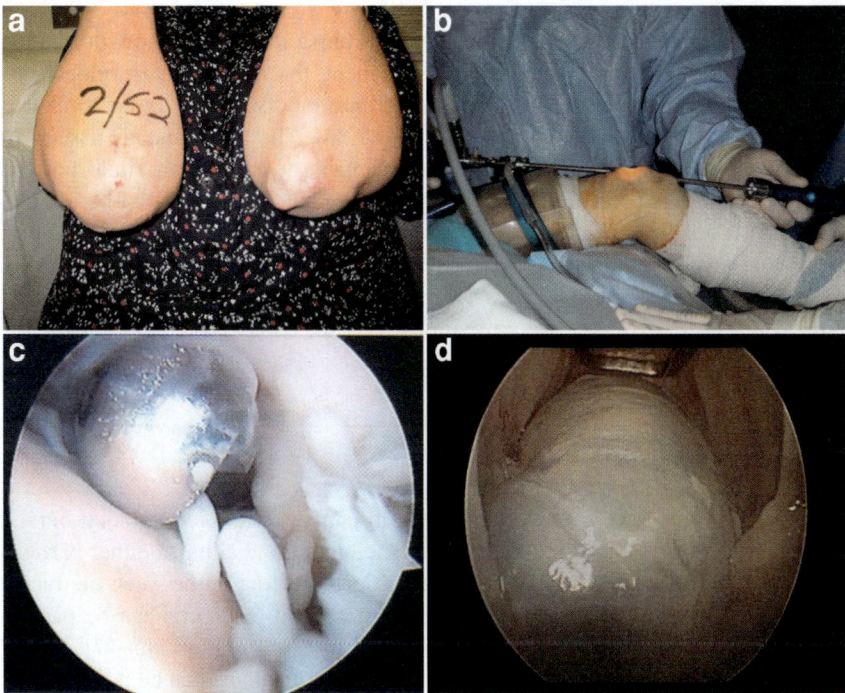

Fig. 7.3 a Bilateral olecranon bursitis. Two weeks following right olecranon endoscopic bursectomy. At least the worst side is now done! **b** Set up for olecranon bursoscopy with wet technique. **c** Olecranon bursoscopy with resector debriding the bursa from in-side out with wet technique. **d** Dry olecranon endoscopy with the hood of the scope seen *above*, which provides a working space so that the bursa can be dissected from the olecranon and subcutaneous tissues, and then removed with a rongeur

technique is now preferred by the authors and involves elevation of the subcutaneous tissues off of the bursa and then resecting the bursa.

7.3.1 Surgical Technique (Wet Technique)

The patient is placed in the lateral decubitus position, with the arm over a padded bolster and a tourniquet around the upper arm (Fig. 7.3b). Two separate 1.5 cm longitudinal portals are made 2 cm proximal and distal to the margins of the bursa, in the midline. Distension is maintained via a gravity feed saline inflow and an arthroscopic cannula that prevent the fluid draining away. The scope can by placed into the bursa and it is then resected from inside out until normal triceps tendon insertion and olecranon are visualised (Fig. 7.3c). Care is required to protect the overlying skin, to prevent any perforations, which can become an irritating sinus.

7.3.2 Surgical Technique (Dry Technique)

The authors' preferred technique of olecranon bursa resection is now dry endoscopy utilising the Stortz endoscopic equipment that has been developed for endoscopic ulnar nerve release [7]. A 2–3 cm incision distal to the bursa is made to allow introduction of the hooded scope (Fig. 7.3d). The subcutaneous tissues are elevated off the bursa and olecranon and then via a separate proximal portal a pituitary rongeur is used to resect the bursa. Rheumatoid nodules can be resected in the same manner. Cautery is used to control bleeding to prevent any fluid accumulation in the bursal space postoperatively.

Previously we have utilised pressure bandages and drains to prevent recurrence of the dead space. However, we now simply have the elbow placed in a sling at 90° of flexion, as this will close off the dead space.

7.4 Distal Biceps Bursoscopy

Bicipitoradial bursoscopy may be indicated in patients with bicipitoradial bursitis or partial tears of the distal biceps tendon. The bicipitoradial bursa either partially or fully envelops the distal biceps tendon to decrease friction between the biceps tendon and the radial tuberosity [15]. The bursitis and tendonitis can be painful, cause radial nerve compression or limitation of forearm rotation [15–17].

Surgery is indicated after failed conservative treatment and can be performed as an open or endoscopic technique. Endoscopy enables a magnified view of the pathology, biopsy and dynamic assessment of the distal biceps [18, 19].

Fig. 7.4 a Setup for distal
biceps bursoscopy.
b Endoscopic view of a
normal cadaveric distal
biceps tendon and bursa.
c Endoscopic view of a
normal cadaveric distal
biceps tendon attaching to the
radius

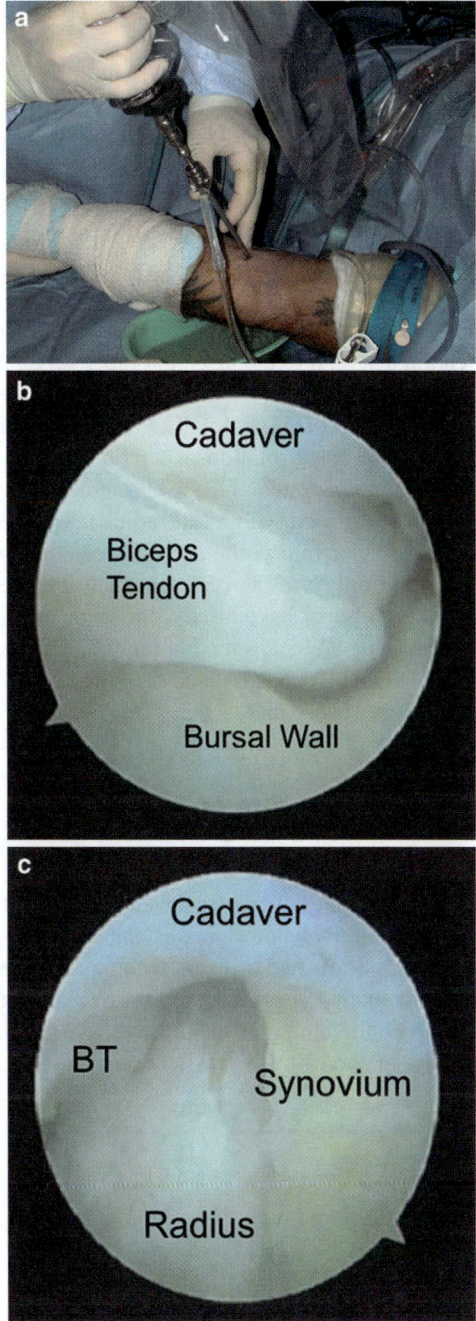

7.4.1 Surgical Technique

The patient is supine with the arm on a table, in extension and supination with a tourniquet applied (Fig. 7.4a). A 2.5 cm longitudinal incision over the biceps tendon, 2 cm distal to the elbow crease is performed, and the lateral cutaneous nerve of the forearm is protected [18–20]. The trochar and arthroscopic cannula are inserted into the bursa on its radial side and normal saline introduced via gravity feed. A pump is not used in order to minimise fluid extravasation into the forearm.

The bursa encircles the two tendons of the distal biceps that are held together by loose areolar tissue, as they approach the insertion (Fig. 7.4b). The long head tendon inserts into the proximal tuberosity and the short head passes anterior to the long head, and inserts in a fan-like manner on the distal portion of the radial tuberosity [21] (Fig. 7.4c). The tendon insertion can be dynamically assessed with a probe, forearm rotation or traction on the tendon with a nylon tape around the more proximal tendon [18]. Debridement of synovitis or a partial tear of the tendon can be performed with a full radius resector with free drainage. Due to the risk of neurovascular injury, the authors' recommend to *not* use suction or resectors with teeth and only use the resector when the aperture is clearly in view.

The authors' have used endoscopy when performing a surgical repair of a complete distal biceps tendon rupture. The anatomic footprint can be identified and debrided endoscopically, and then the tendon repaired to the radial tuberosity as an endoscopic procedure.

7.5 The Future of Endoscopy

Most endoscopy that is performed is wet endoscopy, similar to arthroscopic techniques that have been developed over 40 years. Dry endoscopy of the upper limb is relatively new, but is the area most likely to develop. By using extra working portals and utilising techniques developed in open surgery, we have been able to excise the olecranon bursa, release all the nerves around the elbow, transpose the ulnar nerve, suture the deep fascia, insert suture anchors and perform repairs of the distal biceps tendon.

References

1. Watts AC, Bain GI (2009) Patient-rated outcomes of ulnar nerve decompression: a comparison of endoscopic and open in situ decompression. J Hand Surg Am 34(8):1492–1498
2. Bain GI, Bajhau A (2005) Endoscopic release of the ulnar nerve at the elbow using the Agee device: a cadaveric study. Arthroscopy 21(6):691–695
3. Zlowodzki M, Chan S, Bhandari M, Kalliainen L, Schubert W (2007) Anterior transposition compared with simple decompression for treatment of cubital tunnel syndrome. A meta-analysis of randomized, controlled trials. J Bone Joint Surg Am 89(12):2591–2598

4. Macadam SA, Gandhi R, Bezuhly M, Lefaivre KA (2008) Simple decompression versus anterior subcutaneous and submuscular transposition of the ulnar nerve for cubital tunnel syndrome: a meta-analysis. J Hand Surg Am 33(8):1314 e1–e12
5. Cobb TK, Tyler J, Sterbank P, Lemke J (2008) Efficiency of endoscopic cubital tunnel release. Hand 3:191
6. Cobb TK (2010) Endoscopic cubital tunnel release. J Hand Surg Am 35(10):1690–1697
7. Hoffmann R, Siemionow M (2006) The endoscopic management of cubital tunnel syndrome. J Hand Surg Br 31(1):23–29
8. Tsai TM, Bonczar M, Tsuruta T, Syed SA (1995) A new operative technique: cubital tunnel decompression with endoscopic assistance. Hand Clin 11(1):71–80
9. Pien FD, Ching D, Kim E (1991) Septic bursitis: experience in a community practice. Orthopedics 14(9):981–984
10. Stell IM (1996) Septic and non-septic olecranon bursitis in the accident and emergency department—an approach to management. J Accid Emerg Med 13(5):351–353
11. Ho G Jr, Tice AD, Kaplan SR (1978) Septic bursitis in the prepatellar and olecranon bursae: an analysis of 25 cases. Ann Intern Med 89(1):21–27
12. Fisher RH (1977) Conservative treatment of distended patellar and olecranon bursae. Clin Orthop Relat Res 123:98
13. Ogilvie-Harris DJ, Gilbart M (2000) Endoscopic olecranon bursal resection: the olecranon bursa and prepatellar bursa. Arthroscopy 16(3):249–253
14. Kerr DR, Carpenter CW (1990) Arthroscopic resection of olecranon and prepatellar bursae. Arthroscopy 6(2):86–88
15. Espiga X, Alentorn-Geli E, Lozano C, Cebamanos J (2011) Symptomatic bicipitoradial bursitis: a report of two cases and review of the literature. J Shoulder Eblow Surg 20(2):e5–e9
16. El Hadidi S, Burke FD (1987) Posterior interosseous nerve syndrome caused by a bursa in the vicinity of the elbow. J Hand Surg Br 12(1):23–24
17. Spinner RJ, Lins RE, Collins AJ (1993) Posterior interosseous nerve compression due to an enlarged bicipital bursa confirmed by MRI. J Hand Surg Br 18(6):753–756
18. Bain GI, Johnson LJ, Turner PC (2008) Treatment of partial distal biceps tendon tears. Sports Med Arthrosc. 16(3):154–161
19. Eames MHA, Bain GI (2006) Distal biceps tendon endoscopy and the anterior elbow arthroscopic portal. Tech Shoulder Elbow Surg 7(3):139–142
20. Bain GI, Johnson LJ, Watts AC (2010) Endoscopic distal biceps repair. Chapter 14 in AANA Advanced Arthroscopy, Wrist and Elbow. Saunders-Elsevier
21. Eames MH, Bain GI, Fogg QA, van Riet RP (2007) Distal biceps tendon anatomy: a cadaveric study. J Bone Joint Surg Am 89(5):1044–1049

Arthroscopic Treatment of Elbow Fractures

8

E. Guerra, A. Marinelli, G. Bettelli, M. Cavaciocchi and R. Rotini

8.1 Introduction

Arthroscopy of the elbow is a relatively recent surgical procedure. Although the first experience described in the literature dates back to the 80s, it is only in the last 15 years that a real and increasing interest can be seen with the inclusion of series of patients [1] and case reports that describe the research for new indications.

Intra-articular fractures, by their definition, should be anatomically reduced with extreme accuracy besides being fixed in a stable manner. Arthroscopy has already shown its usefulness in all the joints, by improving the visual field of the joint surface with a minimally-invasive surgical approach.

Besides several case reports in the literature on single fractures, in 2010 Peden et al. [2] performed the first overview on this innovative elbow arthroscopy technique.

The literature shows little scientific evidence about the various indications for arthroscopy of the elbow [3]. These indications include fractures of the radial head, capitellum, trochlea and coronoid.

This chapter addresses the various articular fractures of the elbow, where arthroscopy can nowadays be considered to be a real help. The most important technical aspects are summarized in the light of the literature and the authors' personal experience.

E. Guerra · A. Marinelli · G. Bettelli · M. Cavaciocchi · R. Rotini (✉)
Istituto Ortopedico Rizzoli, Via Delle Rose, 12, 40136 Bologna, BO, Italy
e-mail: roberto.rotini@ior.it

L. A. Pederzini (ed.), *Elbow Arthroscopy,*
DOI: 10.1007/978-3-642-38103-4_8, © ISAKOS 2013

8.2   Fractures of the Capitulum Humeri and Trochlea (Shear Fracture)

Fractures of the capitulum humeri and trochlea are rare fractures that alter the joint considerably. Even when they are not the result of high energy trauma, they produce severe stiffness and instability in the elbow, if they are not immediately recognized and treated adequately [4].

Various classifications try to group the various morphologies and determine correct treatment algorithms [4–7]. Anatomical reduction is necessary to restore the joint anatomy and the correct tension of the external ligament compartment.

8.2.1   In the Literature

Only a few cases have been described. Feldmann [8] reported two cases of fracture with thin osteochondral fragments (Type 2 fracture, Regan and Morrey). Having ascertained the absence of combined joint instability, this author decided for the simple removal of the fragments by arthroscopy using two approaches, antero-medial and anterolateral.

In 2002 Hardy et al. [9] described reduction and fixation of a Hahn-Steinthal fracture (Type I, Regan and Morrey) achieved arthroscopically, by three different anterolateral approaches. The metal screw, in the subchondral bone must be tilted from lateral to medial on the frontal plane, to avoid the radial nerve.

In 2009 Mitani et al. [10] published a new clinical case with interesting practical advice. By two simple anteromedial and anterolateral portals he used the arthroscope together with the probe to reduce the displaced osteochondral fragment; maintaining the reduction with the probe from the anterolateral portal, he performed fixation with two metal screws in a postero-anterior direction.

The following year Kuriyama et al. [11] went a step further by attempting arthroscopic reduction and fixation (ARIF) of two more complex cases (Type IIIA Dubberley) through two portals (anterolateral and midlateral). In one of the two cases the operation was transformed into open surgery, with an incision of only a few centimeters.

8.2.2   Surgical Technique in Our Experience

From 2000 to 2012 about 48 type I or type II shear fractures were treated in our department by open reduction and internal fixation in 43 cases and by miniopen technique in 5 cases. Our experience with arthroscopic treatment started in 2004 with 3 type III fractures in which we performed fragment removal. In the last 2 years our indications were widened to include strictly selected type I and type II fractures (5 cases).

All the patients underwent preoperative CT of the elbow that is essential to define the fracture morphology and to find medial fracture lines directed towards the trochlea or impacted fractures with osteochondral fragments deformity (so-called elbow Hill-Sachs lesions) which can make the reduction more difficult.

In open surgery, the Kocher approach extended proximally (Extensile Kocher approach) with posterolateral subluxation maneuvers, enables easy control over both the anterior articular compartment (with access to the medial trochlea) and the posterior one (to treat impacted lesions).

The capitellum and trochlea fractures that come to our attention are apparently simple injuries. The CT nearly always shows more medial fracture lines (towards the trochlea) or impact lesions with deformation of the osteochondral fragments (elbow Hill Sachs lesions) that make reduction difficult. In arthroscopic surgery, the fracture must be well visualized in the anterior compartment and the posterolateral gutter (Fig. 8.1). Therefore, if arthroscopic treatment is selected, it is not sufficient in our opinion to perform only the anterior or posterolateral portals, but it is necessary to move the arthroscope several times, before performing fixation, which is a very complex procedure.

It is common to find an intraoperative lesion of the external collateral ligament complex, which, in open surgery can be repaired.

Another aspect to take into consideration is the direction of the fixation. We strongly advocate anterograde fixation, with screws and pins made of polylactic acid. In this direction compression fixation can be performed by sinking the screws under the cartilage plane, perpendicularly to the fracture lines. If the ARIF technique is chosen screws that enter posteriorly are needed in order to avoid risks to the radial nerve.

These reasons suggest restricting arthroscopic treatment of capitellum and trochlea fractures to rare cases that fulfill the following criteria:

- Type I fractures (Hahn-Steinthal) without posterior depression
- Type III fractures
- absence of combined ligament lesions

For the recommended surgical technique the patient is placed in a lateral position. Injected sterile saline solution repeatedly to drain the are also recommended. By these three approaches appropriate joint shaving and lesion planning can be performed, by keeping the arthroscope in the medial portals and working through the two lateral portals. Some authors [12, 13] recommend placing the elbow in extension to facilitate reduction. In our opinion, extension reduces the space to work, so we prefer to keep flexion at 90° and operate with the two lateral approaches. After performing temporary reduction and fixation the fracture must be explored posterolaterally. We also recommended exploring the posterior compartment to drain the hematoma and check for any posterior loose bodies (posterolateral and poster central arthroscopic approaches). By the posterolateral portals it will be thus possible to go down posterolaterally to the posterior humeroradial joint (using the palpator and shaver through the midlateral approach). At this point, by bringing the arthroscope back anteromedially under image intensifier

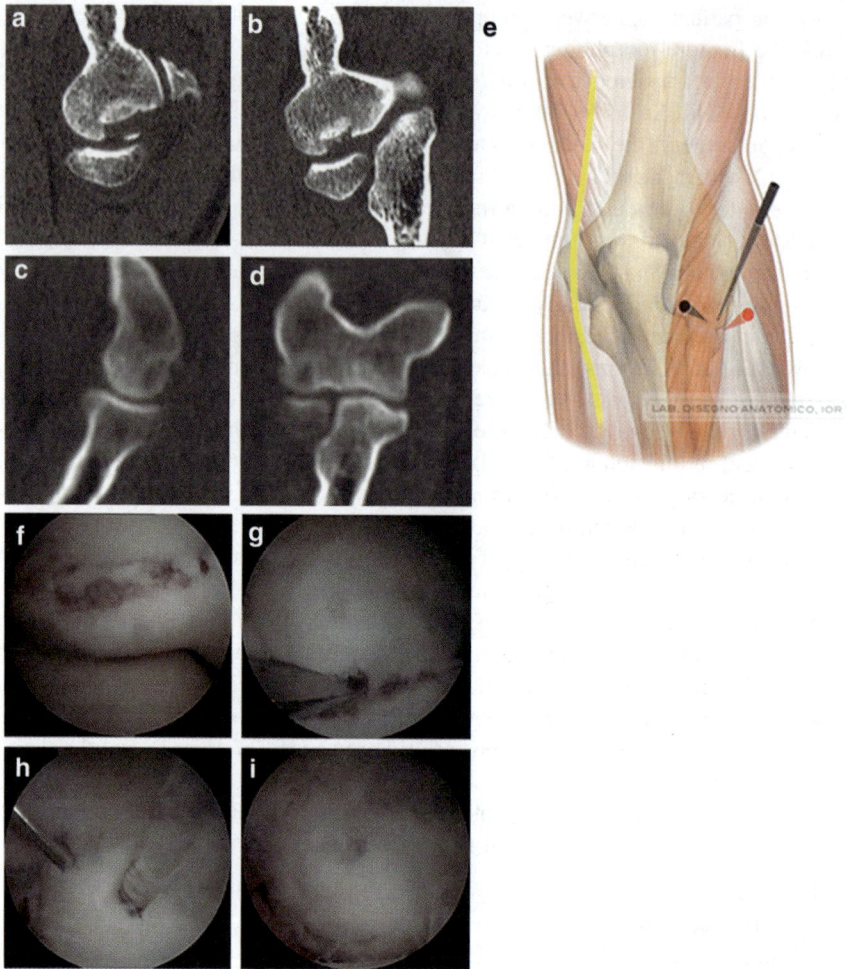

Fig. 8.1 Impacted capitellum fracture. Patient aged 36, *right* elbow. CT scan image of a rare impacted fracture of the posterior face of the capitellum before (**a**, **b**) and after (**c**, **d**) reduction and fixation. Illustration (**e**) of the arthroscopic portals used to perform ARIF of the fracture. Exploration of the anterior joint compartment enabled the tip of the intraarticular fractured coronoid to be removed. In order to see the fracture it was necessary to reach the posterolateral gutter placing the scope in the posterolateral portal (**f**). After reducing the fracture by a probe through the mid-lateral portal (**g**), fixation has been performed by a temporary percutaneous K-wire (**h**) and by a resorbable pin (**h**, **i**) (RSB implant, hit medica, lima corporate)

guidance, percutaneous fixation can be performed with cannulated screws, in a posteroanterior direction (enlarging the midlateral approach).

In our 5 cases, we preferred to end the operation in open surgery, with a small incision that joins the anteromedial portal to the midlateral one (ideally following the incision by the Kocher approach). This miniopen surgery enabled us to perform fixation with resorbable screws and pins, in an anteroposterior direction, without putting the radial nerve at risk.

Treatment was completely arthroscopic with fragments removal in 3 type III cases. Also in these cases we deem mandatory to explore by the arthroscope all the joint compartments, after having accurately examined the fracture comminution by CT scan, in order to reduce the risk of leaving debris.

The last case, apart from the presented series, is a rare impacted fracture of the capitellum combined with a coronoid tip fracture (Fig. 8.1). By arthroscopy it was possible to remove the coronoid fragment (working in the anterior compartment), to raise the impacted osteochondral fragment and fix it with resorbable pins (working in the posterolateral gutter). In this case arthroscopy displayed all of its efficacy, reducing surgical aggressiveness at a minimum.

At the end of fixation or debridement, articular stability is evaluated (possible also arthroscopically [13]). Faced with doubt about the stability, we recommend exploring, and possibly repairing, the lateral collateral ligament.

8.3   Coronoid Fractures

The coronoid plays a key role in elbow joint stability. Fractures were classified into 3 types according to their size by Regan and Morrey [14] in 1989 and only recently have new more complex classifications been devised [15, 16] to include possible morphologies of the fragments connected to the type of injury that can produce them.

Larger fractures are caused by a direct posterior injury, whereas a posterolateral or posteromedial distortion mechanism has been identified for fractures of the apex and medial surface respectively (sublime tubercle insertion site of the anterior bundle of the medial collateral ligament) [16].

Reduction and fixation of coronoid fractures is necessary to restore the anterior and medial elbow stability that was lost with the injury.

When combined with fractures of the radial head, which require prosthetic replacement, after radial head excision the coronoid fracture can be reached through Kocher's lateral approach. Conversely, when the fracture is isolated, reaching and exposing the coronoid requires wide approaches (anterior, antero-medial or medial), which are aggressive and not simple to perform [17].

8.3.1   In the Literature

There are only two articles in the literature

Liu et al. [18] in 1996 showed two cases of coronoid tip fracture, which after conservative treatment produced pain and joint stiffness. Arthroscopic removal of the fracture fragment is decisive.

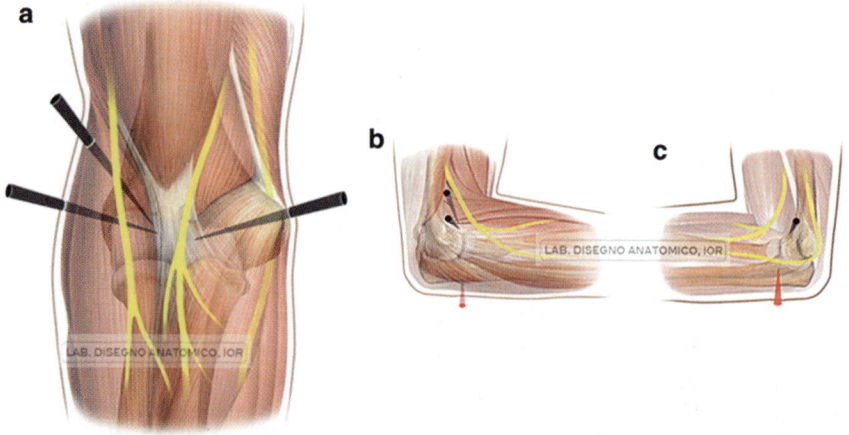

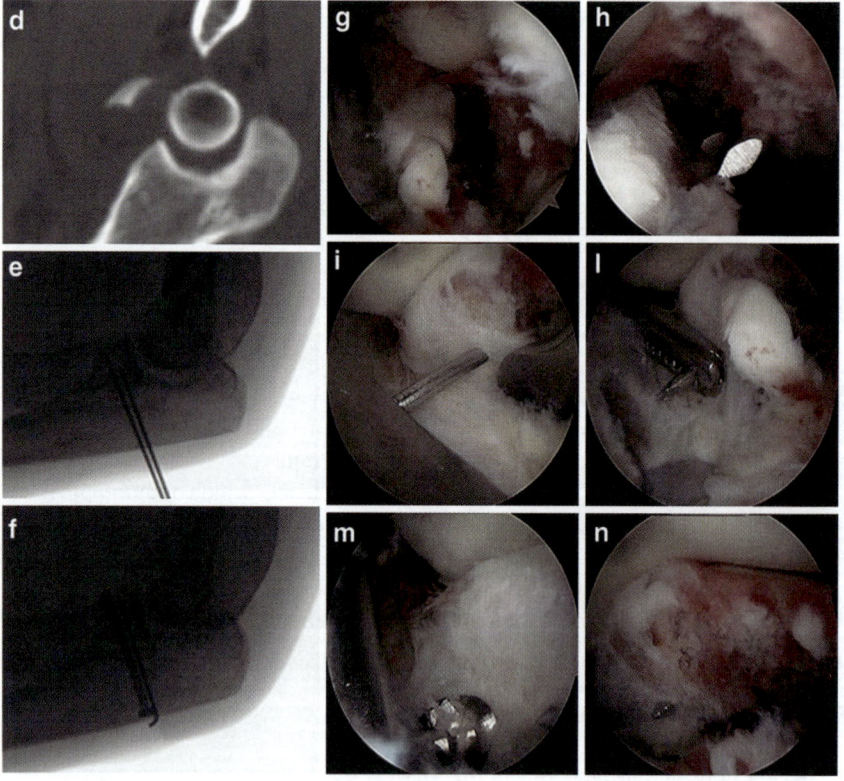

◀ **Fig. 8.2** Coronoid fracture. ARIF of a coronoid fracture: **a**, **b**, **c**—Illustration of the anteromedial, anterolateral and proximal anterolateral arthroscopic portals. *Red* shows the direction of the percutaneous fixation (advisable to perform a small skin incision so as not to interfere with placing the K-wires); **d**—CT scan of the fracture performed routinely to assess the morphology of the fracture and plan surgery; **e**, **f**—intraoperative radiographic checks of the temporary K-wire fixation and definitive fixation with K-wire and cannulated screw; **i**– **n** intraoperative images: with the arthroscope in the anterolateral portal, the retractor in the proximal anterolateral portal and the shaver in the anteromedial one the fracture is exposed (**i**); at least two K-wires are inserted out-in under the fracture fragments (**h**); while keeping the fracture reduced, the wires are pushed forward past the fragment (**h**) protecting the tip (**i**) to avoid lesions to the vascular and neural structures. Depending on the size of the fragments, fixation can be strengthened by placing one or more cannulated screws on the wires (**l**, **m**, **n**)

But the first real experience was described by Adams et al. [19] in 2007. Two of the seven fractures described had fragments that were too small to be fixed. In 4 cases arthroscopically-assisted fixation (ARIF) was performed, whereas in one case open surgery was needed to perform a stronger fixation, by dedicated plate. In 3 of the seven cases reconstruction of the lateral collateral ligament (LUCL) was needed.

8.3.2 Surgical Technique in Our Experience

As for capitellum fractures, coronoid fractures are very rarely isolated. Mostly, they are combined with radial head or olecranon fractures. In these cases, open surgery, necessary to treat combined fractures, cannot be replaced by arthroscopic treatment of the coronoid.

Conversely, isolated fractures of the coronoid can be treated arthroscopically. From January 2000 to July 2012, 5 of the 8 isolated coronoid fractures treated by the authors were treated arthroscopically. Two cases were treated with reduction and fixation with wires alone, two with cannulated screws as well as K wires, and one case with osteosuture combined with K wires.

With the patient in a lateral position, and after having washed repeatedly with needle and saline solution, the anterior arthroscopic portals are made (anteromedial, anterolateral and anteromedial or lateroproximal). Having removed the hematoma the arthroscope is inserted into the anterolateral portal to assess the fracture well. With a motorized instrument and thermal ablator the surfaces of the fragments are exposed. The retractor in the proximal anterior portal (medial or lateral) is fundamental in this phase to keep the joint space open, thus permitting working with a lower inflow pressure. The joint capsule is constantly lacerated and retracted, together with the fragment/s of the fracture. A high pressure of infusion will lead to an early extra-articular swelling, making surgery gradually more difficult and dangerous.

Through the 'combined effect' of the retractor (from the proximal portal) and the probe (from the anteromedial portal) the larger articular fragments are put back in place, thus maintaining the capsular insertion (Fig. 8.2g), whereas the smaller ones can be removed. At this point it is useful to expose the dorsal surface of the ulna with a small incision, so that the skin and the subcutaneous tissue do not interfere with the instruments required for the fixation.

According to the size of the fragments, two different fixation techniques can be used:

- cannulated screws and/or K wires
- osteosuture.

Cannulated screws and/or K wires: (Fig. 8.2). After redislocating the intraarticular fracture with the lever from the proximal portal, K wires are drilled from the posterior cortex of the ulna, keeping the arthroscope in the anterolateral portal and checking its exit from the base of the fractured coronoid (Fig. 8.2h). This action is made safer and repeatable by the use of an aiming device for cruciate ligament surgery; a small-sized tip device must be used, because it has to enter through the anteromedial portal, and a bulky tip might impinge in the brachial muscle. The intraoperative radiographic checking is useful to evaluate the direction of the wires, especially if the freehand technique is chosen.

Having placed the first K wire, the others are placed (at least two to achieve rotational stability of the fixation).

After slightly retracting the wires, until the tip goes into the medullary bone, the fracture is reduced with the lever by the proximal portal, and with an arthroscopic grasper by the anteromedial portal.

While maintaining reduction, the wires are pushed forward again, checking that they come out anteriorly to the fragments (Fig. 8.2i).

When the size of the fragment allows, a cannulated screw, 3.5 mm in diameter, can be placed on one of the K wires. It is cautious to hold the tip of the intra-articular K wire firm with a Kocher, while inserting the cannulated drill and the screw, to prevent the wire from being pushed anteriorly, crossing dangerously the anterior brachial muscle (Fig. 8.2l, m, n).

Osteosuture: this is chosen when the fragments are too small and numerous to be fixed. This fixation will not be as stable as the previous one, but it enables the correct tension of the anteromedial joint capsule to be maintained, while scarring takes place. Often this technique also enables small bone fragments to consolidate.

To contain the joint capsule with suture thread, the suture passer commonly used for suturing rotator cuff lesions is extremely useful (Fig. 8.3d). The work portal is always anteromedial, whereas the arthroscope one remains anterolateral. Once again the retractor through the accessory proximal portal plays a fundamental role.

The vector suture is replaced by a reinforced double-zero suture (Orthocord, Depuy-Mitek or Hi-Fi Conmed Linvatec or Fiberwire Arthrex...) (Fig. 8.3e).

Having placed the suture thread through the joint capsule (immediately behind the fragments of the coronoid tip), the first out-in hole is made at the base of the coronoid with a K wire 1.4 mm in diameter. Having removed the thread, a spinal needle (18 GA 3.50 IN/1.2 * 90 mm spinal needle) (Fig. 8.3f) is inserted by which a vector thread (single-filament 1 mm in diameter), which having been recovered

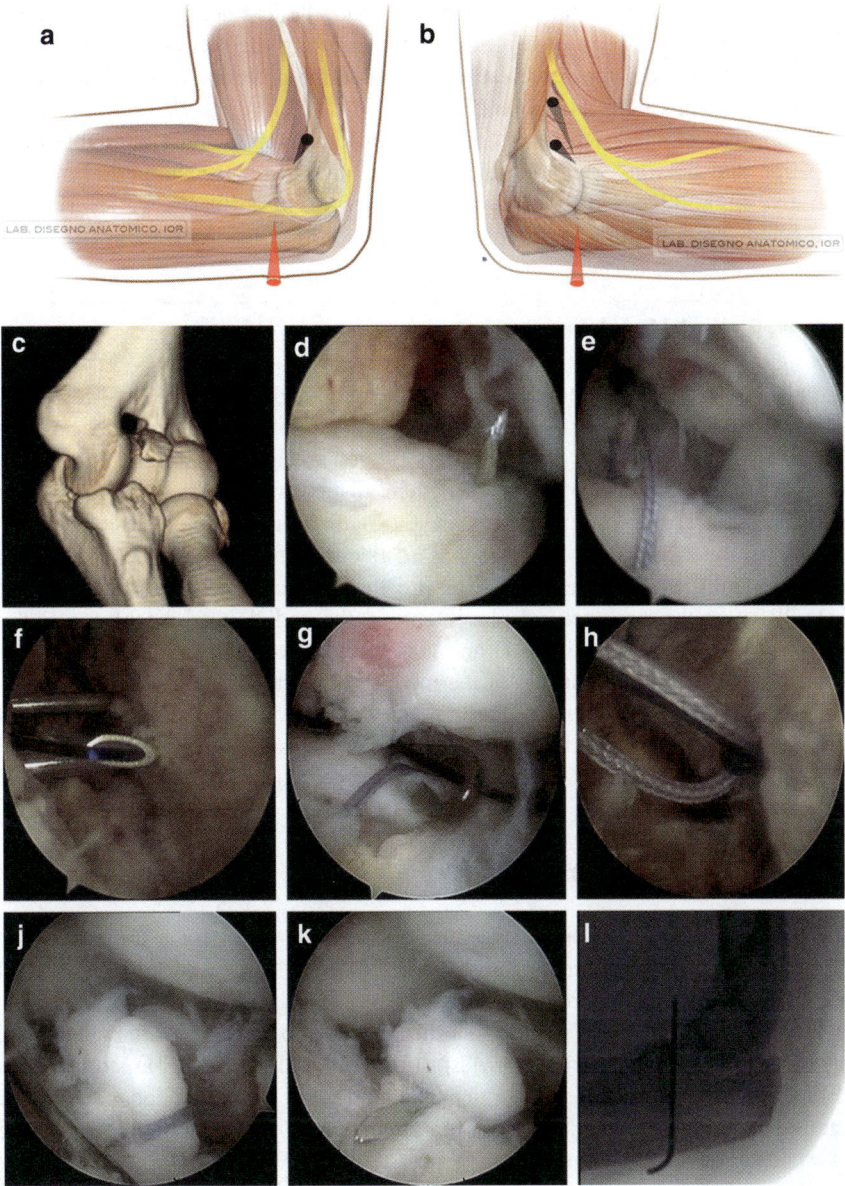

Fig. 8.3 Osteosuture of a coronoid fracture. The portals to perform osteosuture are the same as those used for fixation with K-wires/screws fixation (**a**, **b**). The preoperative CT scan (**c**) shows a displaced fracture. Osteosuture can be performed arthroscopically with the anterolateral arthroscope (**d–k**) as described in the text, possibly reinforced by k_wires (**l**)

from the anteromedial portal (Fig. 8.3g), will take the first head of the osteosuture through the ulna, posteriorly (Fig. 8.3h). By inserting the second head using the same technique, the osteosuture can be closed on the posterior cortex, guiding the fracture fragments with the probe (Fig. 8.3).

Regardless of the ARIF technique chosen, the fixation must be stable upon palpation and flexion–extension tests of the elbow, to reduce the period of postoperative immobilization to a minimum. Therefore, in our cases we always supplemented screw fixation or osteosuture by K wiring (Figs. 8.2f, 8.3k, l).

8.4   Radial Head Fractures

Radial head fractures, extremely common, are classified into 4 types by Mason and Johnston and divided further into simple and complex, according to possible combined lesions [19, 20]. The option of conservative or surgical treatment depends on the number of fragments, their displacement, whether the fracture involves the olecranon and/or coronoid and if there are ligament lesions. When surgery is the choice, the surgeon has to decide among radial head excision, reduction and fixation of the fracture, or prosthetic replacement. It has been shown that ORIF or the prosthetic replacement of the radial head enables a better recovery of articular stability [21] and therefore will certainly be the best choice when there is a combined lesion of the medial collateral ligament. Conversely, an isolated fracture of the radial capitellum can be treated by the simple excision of the fragments (if they interfere with the passive joint range) or by full radial head excision (if more than 50 % of the surface is involved).

8.4.1   In the Literature

The first arthroscopic treatment was described in 2004 [22] for a fracture of the surgical neck of the proximal radius of a child, which was reduced by a manual maneuver and fixed by percutaneous wiring.

In 2006 Rolla et al. [23] published a short series of 6 fractures of the radial head (II, III and IV types according to Mason) reduced and fixed with a percutaneous screw. The author used his own surgical technique, and recommended reducing the fracture by working in the anterior compartment, and moving in the posterolateral gutter for arthroscopic fixation.

Fourteen cases were collected by Michels et al. [24] the following year, all Mason type II with a mean follow-up of 5.6 years and results ranging from good to excellent, matching those of open surgery. For this series the author managed ARIF by the use of only two portals (anterolateral and posterolateral) besides a small incision to insert the screws.

8.4.2 Surgical Technique in Our Experience

In our center arthroscopic treatment of isolated fractures of the radial head began in 2007. Until now 21 cases have been treated arthroscopically (7 ARIF, 8 partial removals of the fragments, 3 radial head excisions and 3 simple reductions, without fixation).

1. *Arthroscopic Reduction Internal Fixation (Arif) for Mason type II fractures*

   The first stage consists of removing the intra-articular hematoma and visualizing the fracture in the anterior compartment. We perform 3 approaches routinely: anteromedial (for the arthroscope) anterolateral (for the tools) and proximal anterolateral (for the retractor). The fracture is reduced by using alternately the probe from the anterolateral portal and proximal anterolateral, by pronosupination movements. Having achieved reduction, the fragments must be stabilized with K wires, after choosing the position in pronosupination to hold for fixation.

   The working position to perform screw fixation may vary. In our experience we divided the fractures according to the position of the fracture fragment/s in relation to the safe zone (part of the radial head that does not come in contact with the small sigmoid notch). Dividing the radial head ideally into two halves in neutral pronosupination we have the lateral half (which contains the Safe Zone) and the medial one (Fig. 8.4).

   Fractures of the lateral half can be fixed by holding the position used for reduction, by placing the forearm in pronation. The retractor and the probe hold reduction and keep the workspace open. An accessory lateral portal is directed at the radial head and a small 5 mm cannula is placed in the joint. The cannula is important to protect the soft tissues from the rotating tools (K wire, drill,

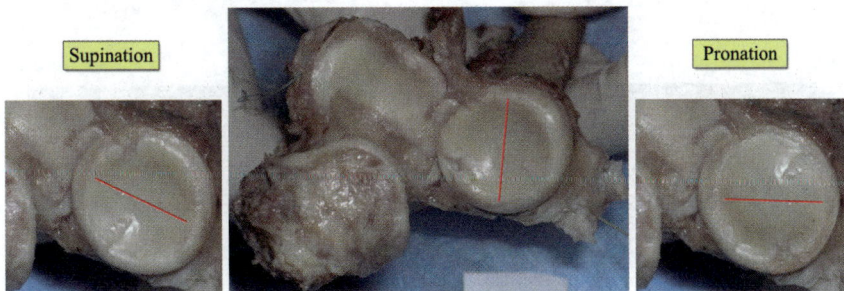

Fig. 8.4 Cadaver specimen. Radial head in full supination, in neutral position and in full pronation. Fractures that involve the half of the radial head opposite to the safe zone, are more difficult to be fixed by the direct lateral portal

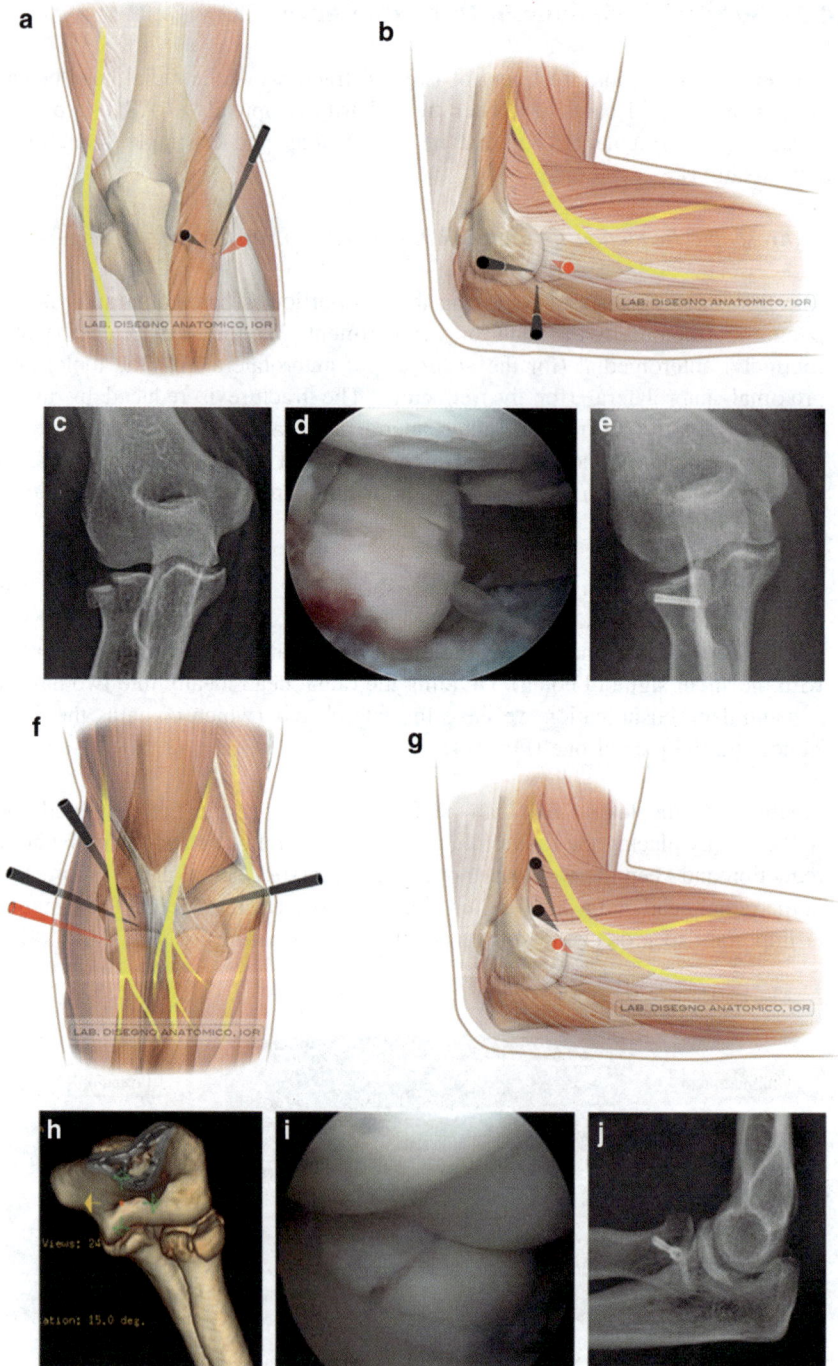

Fig. 8.5 Various fixation methods for radial head fractures: in the posterolateral gutter (**a–e**) and anterior compartment (**f–j**) for radial head fractures that involve the lateral half, fixation is performed through a direct accessory portal (*in red*); in the anterior compartment (**k–r**) for fractures of the medial side of the radial head, fixation is performed through the anteromedial portal (*in red*)

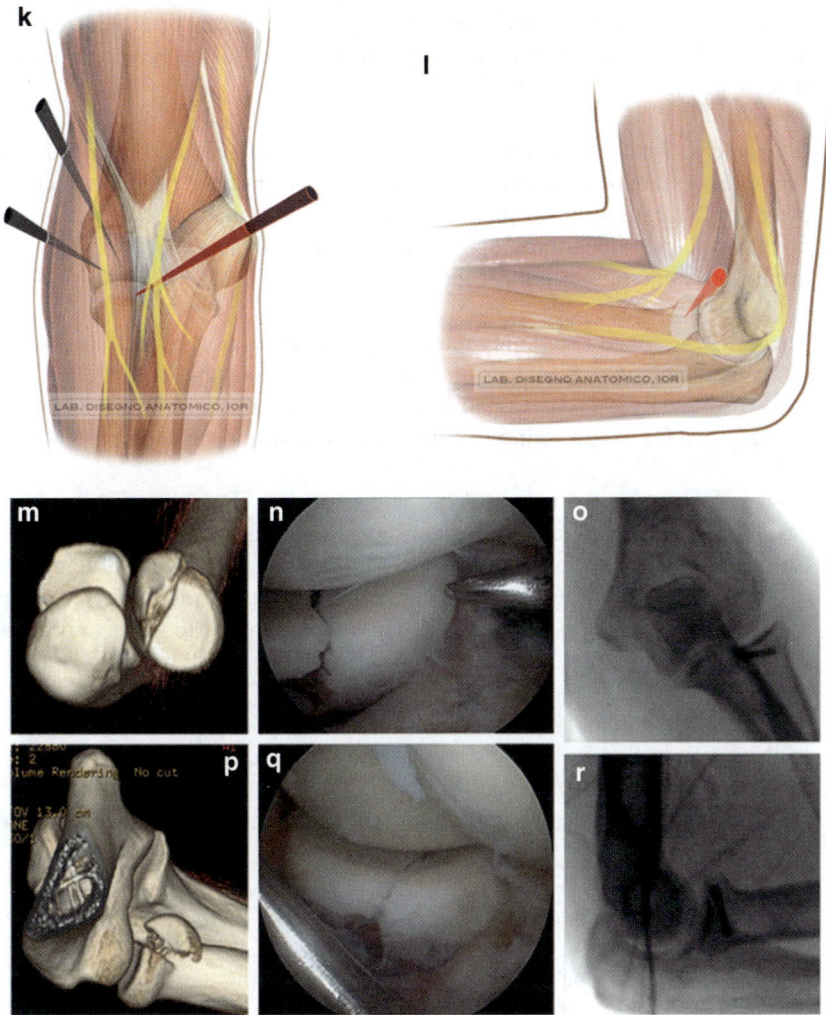

Fig. 8.5 continued

screwdriver) as well as to prevent the thin K wire, used to insert the screw, from bending or breaking. The K wire is inserted through the cannula. If the fracture appears to be stable the fixation procedure is performed (measurement, drilling, screw), otherwise other percutaneous K wires should be placed (outside the cannula) to hold the fragment still while the drill produces the hole for the screw (Fig. 8.5f–j).

Fractures of the lateral half can also be fixed by working in the posterolateral gutter [23] by opening the posterolateral and midlateral portals to place alternately the arthroscope and the work tools. The forearm will have to be progressively placed in supination, until the fracture can be visualized. The procedure for the fixation is the same as that seen in the previous position (Fig. 8.5a–e).

Conversely, when the fracture involves the medial half of the radial head (Fig. 8.5k–r) pronosupination cannot put the fragment to be fixed in the correct place. In this case arthroscopic fixation can be performed by the anteromedial portal by placing the arthroscope in the anterolateral one. The work cannula is even more important to protect the soft tissues.

The ARIF described is certainly more difficult than fixation in open surgery, but offers the numerous advantages of arthroscopy. For example in 4 of the 7 cases treated surgically we found small loose osteochondral fragments not visible by preoperative CT that certainly would not be found in open surgery.

However, choosing the length of the screws is more difficult because it is not easy to perform an intraoperative radiographic check with the tools in place; Generally, the screws range from 14 to 18 mm long and in case of doubt it is better to choose a shorter screw and check at the end of fixation, without risking a loss of reduction or bending the K wires in an attempt to get a satisfactory radiographic view.

The instruments should be chosen carefully so that the drill and the screwdriver of the 2.5 mm diameter screws are not too short, especially when fixation is performed by the anteromedial portal. If these tools are not available, the arthroscopic cannula can be cut on the serving table, before inserting it inside the joint.

2. *Simple Arthroscopic Reduction*

In three cases of Mason fracture type II, after debriding the fracture, reduction was easy. The reduced fragment on the remaining intact part of the radial head was firmly kept in place by the annular ligament, which the arthroscopic technique leaves intact.

After several stability tests we decided to avoid further surgical steps; all cases had a favorable outcome and full, swift recovery.

3. *Arthroscopic Fragment Removal*

In fractures with more comminution, when more than 50 % of the radial head is still in site, fixation is not reliable and prosthetic replacement can be excessive. In these cases, arthroscopic exploration enables removal of the fragments and ample joint debridement, without invalidating articular stability with the

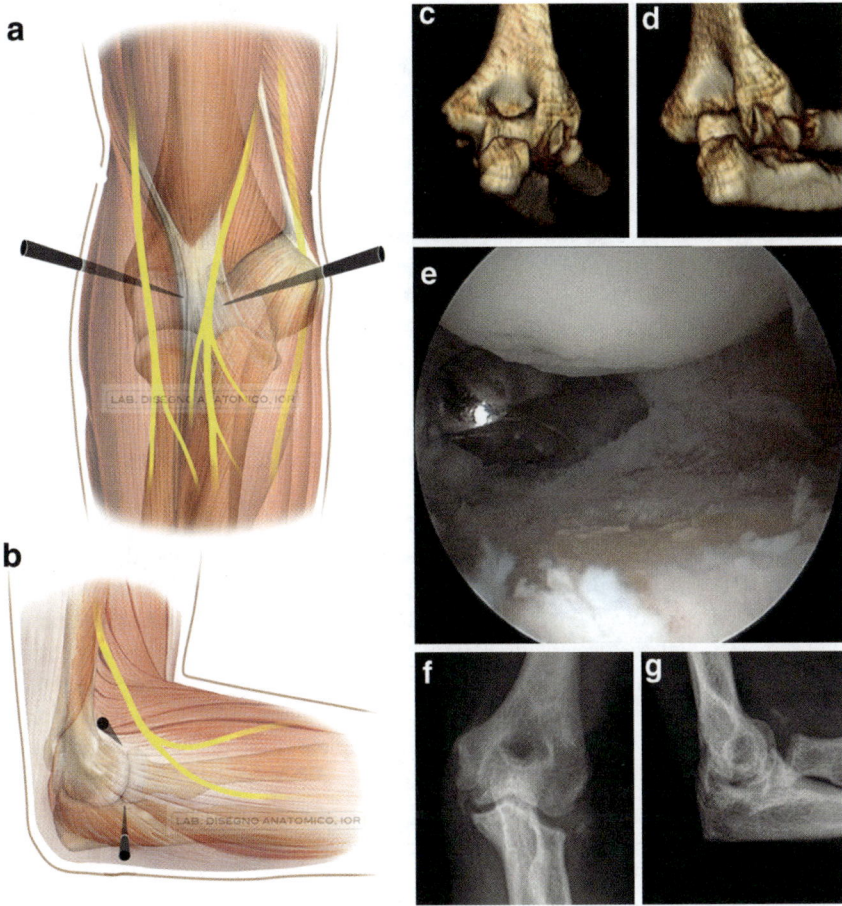

Fig. 8.6 Radial head removal. Illustration (**a, b**) of the anteromedial, anterolateral and midlateral approaches to perform radial head excision; (**c, d**) comminuted fracture of the radial head in an elderly woman where radial head excision is indicated. Intraoperative image (**e**) with the arthroscope in the anteromedial portal monitoring the excision of the radial head performed at the height of the annular ligament by a burr through the midlateral portal. Radiographic check of the radial head excision (**f, g**)

surgical approach. It is performed in the anterior compartment (by anteromedial, anterolateral, and proximal anterolateral approaches) or in the posterolateral gutter (by the posterolateral and midlateral approaches).

Arthroscopy can also be used to assess the articular stability of the ulnohumeral joint [12], which is important in decision-making about radial head prosthesis.

4. *Arthroscopic Radial Head Removal*

When the comminution does not enable fixation, the elbow is stable, and the patient is not so young, resection of the radial head is indicated, which can be performed by arthroscopy.

After removing the fragments in the anterior compartment, resection of the radial head is precise and easy by inserting the burr through the midlateral portal while the arthroscope is still in the anteromedial portal. The radial head is cut at the level of the superior margin of the intact annular ligament. Shortening the proximal radius as little as possible without impairing the annular ligament helps to hold the tension of the lateral collateral compartment (Fig. 8.6).

8.5   Combined Radial Head and Coronoid Fractures

We treated only one case of combined radial head and coronoid fracture arthroscopically. This small-sized radial head fracture was widely displaced; the anterior joint capsule was lacerated and raised with a large fragment of the coronoid. By arthroscopy we followed carefully the path of the radial head fracture, removing the fragments, and performed an ARIF of the coronoid. At the end of the operation the elbow was deemed stable by dynamic tests. Rehabilitation of the patient was begun the day after surgery. Unfortunately, at one-month follow-up, anterior bridge ossifications had formed, with a complete loss of passive movement (Fig. 8.7).

8.6   Complications

No neurological or vascular lesions were recorded.

There were two cases of postoperative stiffness. One Manson II fracture occurred with extension deficit, which was treated again after 9 months by soft tissue release and arthroscopic removal of the screw. The screw was in place, the fracture healed and the stiffness was connected to the reactive fibrosis of the anterior capsule. The soft tissue release enabled the full recovery. The second is the case of heterotopic ossifications as a sequela of the terrible triad treated by arthroscopy.

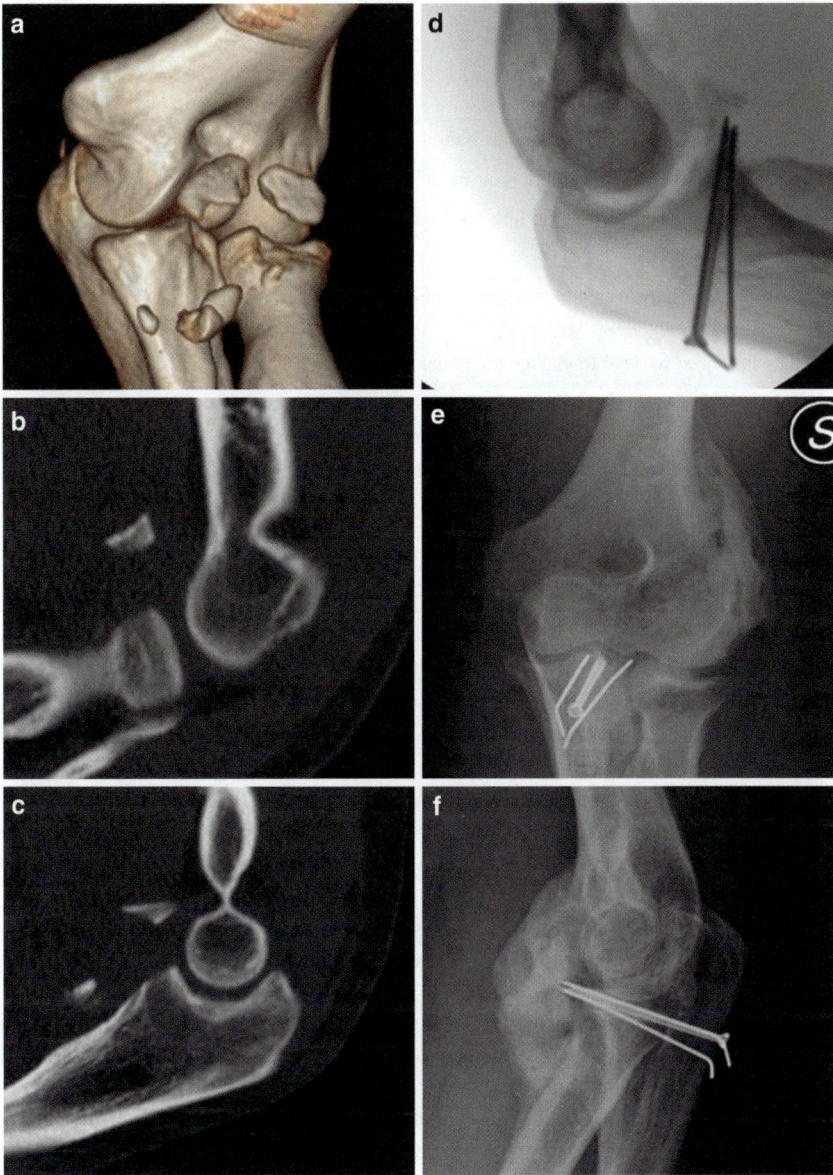

Fig. 8.7 Terrible triad of the *right* elbow in a 28 years old patient. Tridimensional and two-dimensional CT reconstruction (**a, b, c**) of the radial head fracture and coronoid fracture. **d** intraoperative x-ray after arthroscopic removal of the radial head fragments and reduction and internal fixation of the coronoid. **e, f** radiographic follow-up at 4 months shows the massive anterior bridging ossification

Table 8.1 Advantages and limits

Advantages

- Minimally invasive

- Better control of the reduction and stability of the fixation

- Draining of the hematoma and removal of small fragments in the recesses

- Does not preclude conversion into open surgery

Limits

- Current lack of dedicated instruments (aiming device, screwdriver and long cannulated drill, arthroscopic cannulae.

- Possible need to have to change the patient's position if open surgery is required

- Need for precise selection of the surgical indication, excluding beforehand cases that require repair/reconstruction of the collateral ligaments

- Technique still in evolution: although the removal of small articular fragments and radial head excision can also be performed by surgeons with limited experience, conversely ARIF requires deep knowledge of traumatology and of open and arthroscopical elbow surgery.

8.7 Conclusions

The indications for arthroscopic surgery are have become wider and more perfected, over the last two decades, and provide new tools to better address various diseases: one example is the joint fracture treatment which has witnessed the move from surgical debridement to arthroscopic reduction and fixation (ARIF).

The impetus to strive for this difficult but interesting evolution comes from the need to reduce the surgical trauma caused by exposing and reducing articular fractures, which even now give high sequela rates over time.

If 10 years ago ARIF was a future possibility, today it is becoming a reality which, with its advantages and limits (see Table 8.1), is on a par with open surgery.

In this chapter we have tried to summarize the state of the art in the light of our experience. The various surgical techniques described are still not perfectly reproducible, and the surgeon must adapt them to suit each patient. If the feeling is that of a promising road to go down, the two complications that we have highlighted teach us that arthroscopy is also not exempt from the risk of postoperative stiffness. The number of cases is still too small and more in-depth studies are required to assess the real cost/benefit relationship of arthroscopic treatment of articular fractures.

A strict selection of the surgical indication is indispensable; currently we can indicate the following conditions for arthroscopic treatment:

- Fractures of the radial head: Mason type 2–3 fractures (no combined ligament lesions)

- Isolated fractures of the coronoid
- Fractures of the capitulum humeri (no combined ligament lesions)

Only case reports are found for the arthroscopic treatment of combined fractures of the radial capitellum and coronoid, other articular fractures (inter or supracondyloid) or lesions of the lateral collateral ligament [2, 13]. These cases are to be left in the hands of more expert surgeons of the sector, while waiting for further technical development and significant results.

References

1. Kelly EW, Morrey BF, O'Driscoll SW (2001) Complications of elbow arthroscopy. J B J S Am 83:1
2. Peden JP, Savoie FH, Field LD (2010) Arthroscopic treatment of elbow fractures. In: Saunders (ed) The elbow and wrist—AANA advanced artrhoscopy, Chap. 17, pp 136–143
3. Yeoh KM, King GJW, Faber KJ, Glazebrook MA, Athwal GS (2012) Systematic review. Evidence-based indications for elbow arthroscopy. Arthroscopy 28(2):272–282
4. Ring D, Jupiter J, Gulotta L (2003) Articular fractures of the distal part of the humerus. J Bone Joint Surg Am 85:232–238
5. Bryan RS, Morrey BF (1985) Fractures of the distal humerus. In: Morrey BF (ed) The elbow and its disorders. WB Saunders, Philadelphia, pp 325–333
6. McKee MD, Jupiter JB, Bamberger HB (1996) Coronal shear fractures of the distal end of the humerus. J Bone Joint Surg Am 78:49–54
7. Dubberley JH, Faber KJ, Macdermid JC, Patterson SD, King GJ (2006) Outcome after open reduction and internal fixation of capitellar and trochlear fractures. J Bone Joint Surg Am 88(1):46–54
8. Feldman MD (1997) Arthroscopic excision of type II capitellar fractures. Arthroscopy 13(6):743–748
9. Hardy P, Menguy F, Guillot S (2002) Arthroscopic treatment of capitellum fracture of the humerus. Arthroscopy 18(4):422–426
10. Mitani M, Nabeshima Y, Ozaki A, Mori H, Issei N, Fujii H, Fujioka H, Doita M (2009) Arthroscopic reduction and percutaneous cannulated screw fixation of a capitellar fracture of the humerus: a case report. J Shoulder Elbow Surg 18(2):e6–e9 Epub 2008 Nov 25
11. Kuriyama K, Kawanishi Y, Yamamoto K (2010) Arthroscopic-assisted reduction and percutaneous fixation for coronal shear fractures of the distal humerus: report of two cases. J Hand Surg Am 35(9):1506–1509 Epub 2010 Aug 21
12. Hsu JW, Gould JL (2009) The emerging role of elbow arthroscopy in chronic use injuries and fracture care. Hand Clin 25:305–321
13. Holt MS, Savoie FH III, Field LD, Ramsey JR (2004) Arthroscopic management of elbow trauma. Hand Clin 20:485–495
14. Regan NM, Morrey BF (1992) Classification and treatment of coronoid process fractures. Orthopaedics 15(7):345–353
15. O'Driscoll SW, Jupiter JB, Cohen MS, Ring D, McKee MG (2003) Difficult elbow fractures: pearls and pitfalls. Instuc Course Lect 52:113–134
16. Pollock JW, Brownhill J, Ferreira L, McDonald CP, Johnson J, King GJW (2009) The effect of anteromedial facet fractures of the coronoid and lateral collateral ligament injury on elbow stability and kinematics. J Bone Joint Surg Am 91(6):1448–1458
17. Cheung EV, Steinmann SP (2009) Surgical approaches to the elbow. Am Acad Orthop Surg 17:325–333

18. Liu SH, Henry M, Bowen R (1996) Complications of type I coronoid fractures in competitive athletes: report of two cases and review of the literature. J Shoulder Elbow Surg 5(3):223–227
19. Adams JE, Merten SM, Steinmann SP (2007) Arthroscopic-assisted treatment of coronoid fractures. Arthroscopy 23(10):1060–1065
20. Van Riet RP, Van Glabbeek F, Morrey BF (2009) Radial head fracture. In: Morrey BF (ed) The elbow and its disorders, 4th edn. Saunders Elsevier, Philadelphia, PA, pp 359–381
21. Pike JM, Athwal GS, Faber KJ, King GJW (2009) Radial head fractures-an update. J Hand Surg 34A:557–565
22. Dawson FA, Inostroza F (2004) Arthroscopic reduction and percutaneous fixation of a radial neck fracture in a child. Arthroscopy 20(Suppl 2):90–93
23. Rolla PR, Surace MF, Bini A, Pilato G (2006) Arthroscopic treatment of fractures of the radial head. Arthroscopy 22(2):233.e1–233.e6
24. Michels F, Pouliart N, Handelberg F (2007) Arthroscopic management of Mason type 2 radial head fractures. Knee Surg Sports Traumatol Arthrosc 15(10):1244–1250 Epub 2007 Jul 17

Elbow Arthroscopy Complications

9

Graham J. W. King

9.1 Introduction

As techniques evolve and indications expand, arthroscopy has become a mainstay in the treatment of a variety of intra and peri-articular elbow pathologies. Successful outcomes can be achieved safely, but one must be cognisant of the pitfalls associated with this intervention. This chapter provides an overview of the common and rare complications associated with elbow arthroscopy, and steps that may be taken to mitigate risk and avoid misadventure.

9.2 Neurologic Injury

One of the most serious complications of elbow arthroscopy is nerve injury, which has been reported in all forms from neuropraxic to neurotemetic damage. The reported prevalence of neurologic injury in the literature is 0–14 % depending on the series and indication; fortunately most are transient phenomena [1, 2]. Nerve injury can occur secondary to compression or direct injury from instruments, excessive joint distension, aggressive manipulation or post-operative CPM [1]. Local anaesthetic blocks are commonly used for postoperative pain control with elbow arthroscopy including intra-articular injections, regional brachial plexus blocks and cutaneous infiltration around portal sites. Local anesthetic can cause transient nerve palsies, which prevents the post-operative evaluation of nerve function until the effect has resolved; therefore its use has been discouraged by some authors [1, 3, 4]. Unfortunately, more significant partial or complete nerve damage can also occur, and may be caused by direct trauma from portal creation or

G. J. W. King (✉)
University of Western Ontario St Josephs Health Centre, 268 Grosvenor Street, London, ON N6A 4L6, Canada
e-mail: gking@uwo.ca

L. A. Pederzini (ed.), *Elbow Arthroscopy*,
DOI: 10.1007/978-3-642-38103-4_9, © ISAKOS 2013

as a consequence of mechanical or thermal injury from arthroscopic instruments. There are nerve-specific risks inherent to each portal used for elbow arthroscopy, and these are detailed below.

Cutaneous nerve damage is possible during portal creation, and has been described for the medial antebrachial cutaneous nerve [1, 5, 6], and superficial radial nerve [1, 6, 7]. These injuries may be minimized during portal placement by incising only the dermis in line with the arm, then using a blunt instrument such as a haemostat to spread the subcutaneous and fascial tissues down to and through the capsule [8].

Care should be taken during portal placement as multiple previous anatomic studies have documented the close proximity of the surrounding neurovascular structures [5, 9, 10]. During arthroscopy of the anterior compartment of the elbow, the posterior interosseous branch of the radial nerve and median nerve are at risk, and may be as close as 6 mm to the capsule [9]. The elbow should be insufflated with fluid to distend the capsule and displace the neurovascular structures away from the articulation. This increases the bone to nerve distance and working space, reducing the risk of nerve damage when the arthroscopy instruments are introduced into the joint [5]. Despite this step, the limited distance between the capsule and neurovascular structures does not change making nerve injury a constant risk while using instruments within the joint [10]. The portal to nerve distance is increased by keeping the elbow in 90° of flexion and with more proximal anteromedial and anterolateral portals [9–13]. The authors use a small caliber blunt switching stick to palpate the joint, and once satisfied that the instrument is intraarticular, the arthroscopy trocar is introduced over the switching stick and into the joint to avoid extra-capsular insertion [4].

Switching sticks and cannulas should be used to reduce the risk of insertional nerve damage while changing portals. Every attempt should be made to maintain an intact capsule while working in the elbow. On the radiocapitellar side, the posterior interosseous nerve is located subjacent to the anterior capsule along the radial neck. It is at risk of transient neuropraxia from pressure if the portal is placed too far anterior and/or distal to the lateral epicondyle [14, 15]. The posterior interosseous nerve is protected by introducing the trocar over a switching stick with the elbow flexed to 90°, the forearm pronated and the joint insufflated. Care should be taken when resecting any synovitis, radiocapitellar plicae or capsule anterior to the radial head. The posterior interosseous nerve can be damaged or transected by suction shavers, mechanical punches or electrocautery probes [16, 17]. Electrocautery instruments should be insulated and unidirectional, as unintentional heat transfer into the non-targeted tissue can result in neurologic injury [18]. Cautery should be used only in short sequential bursts to allow for heat dissipation in the arthroscopic effluent. A proximal anterolateral portal is used 2 cm proximal and 1 cm anterior to the lateral epicondyle because it is farther from the posterior interosseous nerve and hence is safer than a more distal anterolateral portal [11, 13]. A mid-anterolateral portal can also be employed in the setting where multiple anterolateral portals are required, such as when a retractor is utilized. This is usually made with an inside-out technique using a sharp switching stick.

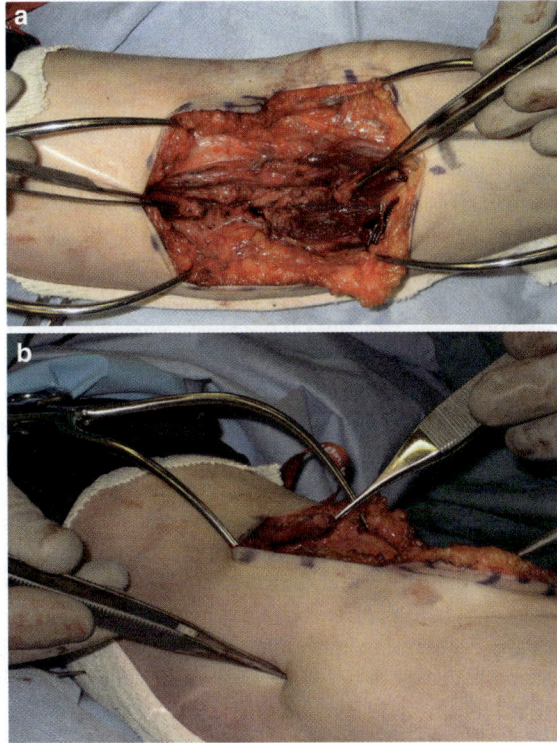

Fig. 9.1 **a** Depicts a neurotemetic median nerve injury after arthroscopic contracture release in a 19 year old male who had previously sustained a simple elbow dislocation. Note the deficient brachial is putting the median nerve at risk. **b** Demonstrates the proximity of the nerve relative to the proximal anteromedial portal. Cable grafting with sural nerve was required for reconstruction

Transient neuropraxia of the anterior interosseous nerve [19] and median nerve have been reported, the latter after removal of large loose bodies through the proximal anteromedial portal [20]. Direct injury to the median and ulnar nerves has also been reported with similar mechanisms to that described for the posterior interosseous nerve. Strategies to protect the median nerve at the anterior aspect of the elbow are similar to those used for the posterior interosseous nerve. The authors use a proximal anteromedial portal 1 cm proximal and 1 cm anterior to the medial epicondyle, avoiding distal portal placement. Cannulas should be used, and the elbow should be kept in a position of flexion. When debriding synovitis, osteophytes, adhesions etc. in the anterior ulnohumeral region, the operator must take care not to perforate the capsule as both anterior interosseous nerve [21] and median nerve injury can occur directly [9]. As with the lateral side, a mid-anteromedial portal can be made with an inside-out technique and used as an accessory portal for retractors if needed (Fig. 9.1).

When transitioning to arthroscopy of the posterior compartment, cannulas are ideally removed from the anterior portals. In many circumstances during posterior arthroscopy the elbow is brought into extension to protect the trochlear cartilage and allow osteophyte removal from the olecranon. Elbow extension can cause a pressure phenomenon between the radial and median nerves and anterior cannula, predisposing to neuropraxia [10]. Frequently, the authors leave a drainage cannula in the proximal anteromedial portal during posterior arthroscopy, as the median nerve seems less predisposed to this complication. Full elbow extension should be avoided however, until all anterior cannulae are removed.

Damage to the ulnar nerve can occur in a variety of situations. It is imperative that the surgeon be aware of ulnar nerve hypermobility and subluxation, which can predispose to contusion or laceration when creating anteromedial portals. Iatrogenic injury can also occur if portals are created blindly after a subcutaneous ulnar nerve transposition has occurred [22]. Subluxation or prior transposition was previously thought to be a relative contraindication to elbow arthroscopy, but some authors have presented strategies for the experienced elbow arthroscopic to mitigate the risk of direct trauma [23]. The subluxation ulnar nerve can be held in a reduced position behind the medial epicondyle while a proximal anteromedial portal is created and a switching stick is inserted into the joint. In the setting of a prior transposition, the location of the ulnar nerve may be unclear. If the nerve position is palpable, then the authors suggest a 1 cm incision and blunt dissection to the capsule without identification. Conversely, if the location of the ulnar nerve is impossible to discern, then a 2–4 cm incision should be made, the nerve identified and protected, and only then should a capsular portal be created [23] (Fig. 9.2).

Even when located in the groove however, the ulnar nerve can be injured with proximal anteromedial portals that are placed over 2 cm proximal to the medial epicondyle, where the ulnar nerve loses its protection from the medial intermuscular septum [24]. The ulnar nerve is most at risk during debridement of the medial gutter when performing posterior compartment arthroscopy. Neurotemetic injury has been described just proximal to the cubital tunnel [25, 26] and for this reason, the authors do not use suction and debride the medial gutter with extreme caution. The instruments are hooded and face away from the ulnar nerve at all times, keeping the adjacent capsule intact. While arthroscopic in situ ulnar nerve decompression has been described, the safety and efficacy has not yet been established [27]. Advanced skills with elbow arthroscopy as well as experience with this procedure in cadavers are recommended prior to performing arthroscopic ulnar nerve decompression in patients.

As the anatomy of the elbow becomes progressively more distorted, particularly in the scenario of rheumatoid arthritis or post-traumatic contractures, the risks of neurologic injury become higher [1]. Expert arthroscopists have suggested guidelines for elbow arthroscopy indications that are stratified by the operator's level of experience [28]. Contracture release should only be attempted in experienced hands and a cautionary account exists of multiple neurotemetic injuries following attempted release in suboptimal conditions [29]. In the setting of arthroscopic rheumatoid synovectomy, debridement should occur cautiously in the anterior compartment with intra-articular retractors, as the capsule is thin and fails to function well as a protective layer for both the median and posterior interosseous nerves [4, 21]. Arthroscopists who choose to incorporate contracture release

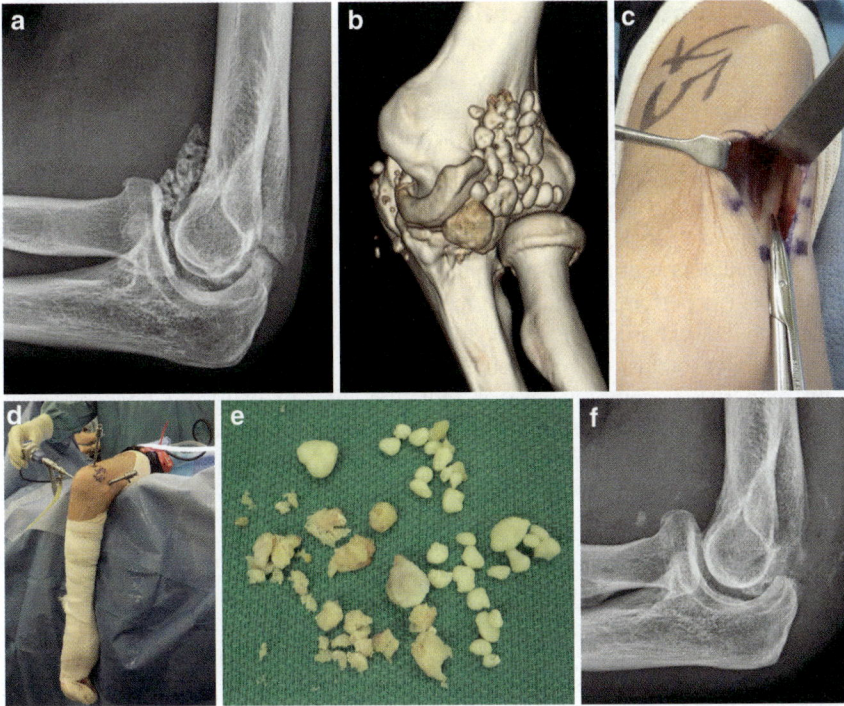

Fig. 9.2 a Depicts the lateral radiograph of a 49 year old male with symptomatic elbow osteoarthritis, loose bodies and an associated ulnar neuropathy. **b** A 3D CT reconstruction of the same elbow. **c** An in situ ulnar nerve decompression is performed prior to elbow arthroscopy for intra-articular debridement and the removal of loose bodies. **d** Demonstrates the proximal anteromedial and anterolateral portals with a posterior central drainage portal relative to the in situ ulnar nerve decompression site. **e** Loose bodies and osteophyte fragments removed during the arthroscopic elbow debridement. **f** A lateral post-operative radiograph demonstrating successful debridement of the osteophytes and loose bodies

into their armamentarium should begin by releasing capsule directly off bone on the humeral side [9] as the neurologic structures may be scarred to capsule anteriorly. As the operator's skill level advances, they may consider incising the capsule across its width. To perform this safely, a duckbill basket punch is used to create a capsular window. Brachial is then visualized and dissected with the anterior neurovascular structures off capsule. Once they are safely palpated and identified, then remainder of the capsule can then be incised [1]. Finally, experienced arthroscopists may choose the technique of endoscopic extracapsular capsulectomy, which permits a more aggressive capsular excision while using retractors to maintain the radial and median nerves at a safe distance [1].

9.3   Heterotopic Ossification

Another risk with elbow arthroscopy is the development of heterotopic ossification post-operatively [30–34]. This can present as a spectrum, from scattered asymptomatic deposition in the surrounding soft tissues [30] to disabling ankylosis requiring open resection [31–34]. Reported risk factors for the development of heterotopic ossification include recent prior surgery, a past history of HO, associated burns and trauma, diffuse skeletal hyperostosis (DISH), CNS pathology and abnormalities of BMP metabolism [33]. The authors routinely use prophylaxis against HO when significant osseous debridement is performed and if no medical contraindications exist. Indomethacin (25 mg po TID) is used for 3 weeks post-operatively in conjunction with a proton pump inhibitor for gastric protection (Fig. 9.3).

In high risk patients, a dose of radiation therapy may also be considered, however since the incidence of significant HO is unknown and likely low we have not employed radiation for primary prophylaxis. We assess patients radiographically 6 weeks postoperatively for signs of HO and modulate their physiotherapy accordingly if present.

9.4   Infection

Like all surgery, there exists a risk for superficial and deep infection with elbow arthroscopy. Multiple authors have reported cases of prolonged drainage from portal sites and/or cellulitis which have resolved with oral antibiotic therapy [1, 4, 26, 35–38]. Unfortunately, there have also been circumstances where deep infection has occurred, in some cases requiring further surgical irrigation and debridement for control [1, 39]. There is an association between the development of a deep infection and arthroscopy with a concurrent intra-articular steroid injection; consequently steroids should be avoided [1]. The authors routinely administer a single dose of intravenous antibiotics prior to arthroscopic elbow surgery.

9.5   Post-Operative Contracture

Recalcitrant elbow stiffness can occur after arthroscopy. The risk seems highest with surgery for post-traumatic disorders of the elbow, including arthroscopic contracture release and arthroscopic-assisted intervention for fracture [1, 4, 40–43]. Often, post-arthroscopy stiffness will respond to active, active-assisted and passive range of motion exercises, as well as a splinting regimen. The authors routinely use a flexion cuff and night-time extension splint to help regain terminal flexion-extension in such circumstances. Static progressive splinting using a turnbuckle may also be employed as an adjunct if progress is slow or plateaus. Unfortunately, in rare circumstances re-operation is necessary for revision contracture release [40, 42–44] and the risk of this seems higher when there are

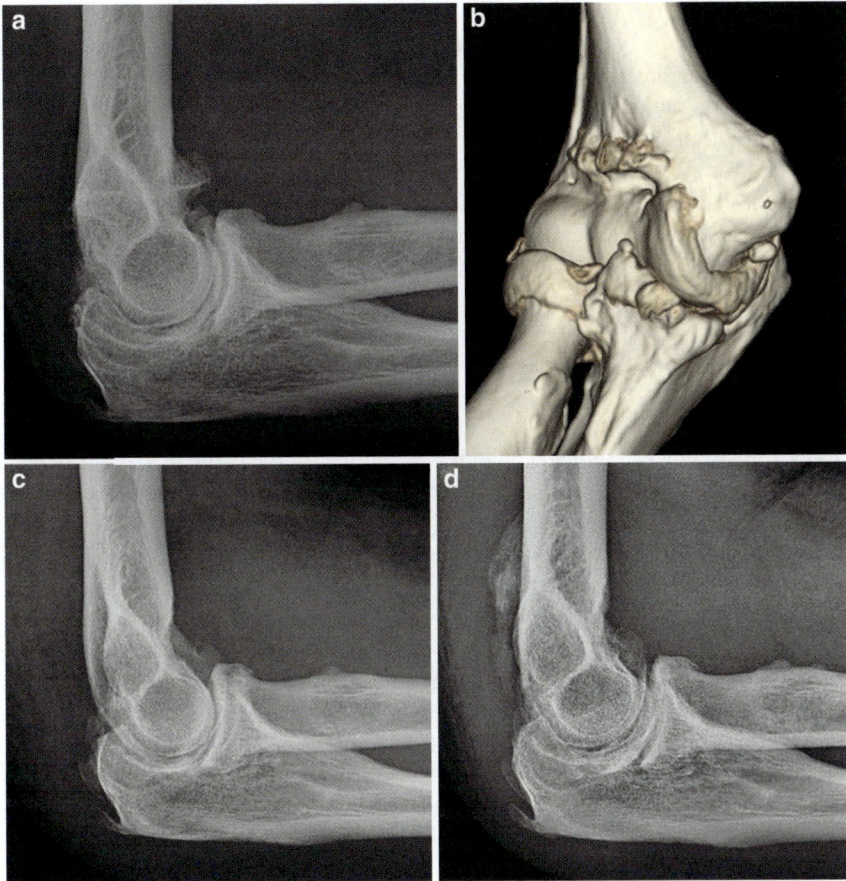

Fig. 9.3 a A lateral radiograph depicting elbow osteoarthritis in a 74 year old male with impingement symptoms. **b** A 3D CT reconstruction of the same elbow. **c** A lateral radiograph taken 10 days post arthroscopy demonstrating successful debridement of the osteophytes and loose bodies. **d** A lateral radiograph taken 6 weeks post-operatively depicting heterotopic ossification along the posterior aspect of the humerus. No prophylaxis had been given because of the risk of GI ulceration

associated degenerative joint changes, possibly due to articular pain limiting motion during rehabilitation [42, 43].

9.6 Uncommon Complications

Other more rare and unusual complications have been reported with elbow arthroscopy. A retained loose body can occur, with symptoms of residual catching or locking [6]. The likelihood of this is much higher if unicompartmental arthroscopy is performed. Thus, both the anterior, posterior and lateral compartments should routinely be evaluated if the intervention is primarily for loose body removal. The medial and lateral gutters are common locations for loose bodies to be missed. The number of loose bodies also plays a role, and patients should be counselled of this risk accordingly, particularly if elbow arthroscopy is being performed for synovial osteochondromatosis where hundreds of loose bodies may be present. Hematoma formation has been described, but is a rarely reported sequela [38]. Lastly, subcutaneous emphysema has occurred after elbow arthroscopy, and may be attributable to post-operative drain use or enlarged portals in conjunction with early range of motion exercises [45].

9.7   Conclusion

Elbow arthroscopy is a safe and effective technique for the surgical management of a variety of intra and peri-articular pathologies. Potential complications exist, but their risk of occurrence can be mitigated by the strategies presented in this article. In particular, the anteromedial and anterolateral portals should be made proximal to the epicondyles to reduce the risk of iatrogenic nerve injury. Anterior portals should be made with the elbow flexed, insufflated with sterile fluid, and for the lateral side with the elbow in pronation. A narrow caliber switching stick should be the first instrument placed in the joint to reduce the risk of extra-capsular insertion. Inflow of fluid into the joint should be gravity fed or under low pressure if a pump is used, to prevent over distension, and an outflow cannula should be used for drainage. Electrocautery devices should be used cautiously and on only for short bursts. Retractors should be used liberally in the anterior compartment, and the capsule should be left intact when possible to reduce the risk of nerve injury. Posteriorly, debridement in the medial gutter should be cautiously performed and without suction to prevent iatrogenic ulnar nerve trauma. Most important of all, surgeons should move slowly up the arthroscopic skill ladder, advancing to complicated indications only once sufficient experience has been attained with simpler procedures.

References

1. Kelly EW, Morrey BF, O'Driscoll SW (2001) Complications of elbow arthroscopy. J Bone Joint Surg Am 83-A(1):25–34
2. Lattermann C, Romeo AA, Anbari A, Meininger AK, McCarty LP, Cole BJ, Cohen MS (2010) Arthroscopic debridement of the extensor carpi radialis brevis for recalcitrant lateral epicondylitis. J Shoulder Elbow Surg 19:651–656
3. Andrews JR, Carson WG (1985) Arthroscopy of the elbow. Arthroscopy 1:97–107
4. O'Driscoll SW, Morrey BF (1992) Arthroscopy of the elbow: diagnostic and therapeutic benefits and hazards. J Bone Joint Surg Am 74:84–94
5. Lynch GJ, Meyers JF, Whipple TL, Caspari RB (1986) Neurovascular anatomy and elbow arthroscopy: inherent risks. Arthroscopy 2(3):190–197

6. Ogilvie-Harris DJ, Schemitsch E (1993) Arthroscopy of the elbow for removal of loose bodies. Arthroscopy 9:5–8
7. Guhl JF (1985) Arthroscopy and arthroscopic surgery of the elbow. Orthopedics 8(10):1290–1296
8. Marshall PD, Fairclough JA, Johnson SR, Evans EJ (1993) Avoiding nerve damage during elbow arthroscopy. J Bone Joint Surg—Brit Volume 75(1):129–131
9. Miller C, Jobe C, Wright M (1995) Neuroanatomy in elbow arthroscopy. J Shoulder Elbow Surg 4(3):168–174
10. Unlu M, Kesmezacar H, Akgun I, Ogut T, Uzun I (2006) Anatomic relationship between elbow arthroscopy portals and neurovascular structures in different elbow and forearm positions. J Shoulder Elbow Surg 15(4):457–462
11. Field LD, Altchek DW, Warren RF, O'Brien SJ, Skyhar MJ, Wickiewicz TL (1994) Arthroscopic anatomy of the lateral elbow: a comparison of three portals. Arthroscopy 10(6):602–607
12. Lindenfeld TN (1990) Medial approach in elbow arthroscopy. Am J Sports Med 18(4):413–417
13. Stothers K, Day B, Regan WR (1995) Arthroscopy of the elbow: anatomy, portal sites, and a description of the proximal lateral portal. Arthroscopy 11(4):449–457
14. Papilion JD, Neff RS, Shall LM (1988) Compression neuropathy of the radial nerve as a complication of elbow arthroscopy: a case report and review of the literature. Arthroscopy 4(4):284–286
15. Thomas MA, Fast A, Shapiro D (1987) Radial nerve damage as a complication of elbow arthroscopy. Clin Orthop Relat Res 215:130–131
16. Gupta A, Sunil TM (2004) Complete division of the posterior interosseous nerve after elbow arthroscopy: a case report. J Shoulder Elbow Surg 13(5):566–567
17. Jones GS, Savoie FH 3rd (1993) Arthroscopic capsular release of flexion contractures (arthrofibrosis) of the elbow. Arthroscopy 9(3):277–283
18. Park JY, Cho CH, Choi JH, Lee ST, Kang CH (2007) Radial nerve palsy after arthroscopic anterior capsular release for degenerative elbow contracture. Arthroscopy 23 (12):1360. e1–1360.e3
19. Salini V, Palmieri D, Colucci C, Croce G, Castellani ML, Orso CA (2006) Arthroscopic treatment of post-traumatic elbow stiffness. J Sports Med Phys Fitness 46:99–103
20. Kim SJ, Kim HK, Lee JW (1995) Arthroscopy for limitation of motion of the elbow. Arthroscopy 11:680–683
21. Ruch DS, Poehling GG (1997) Anterior interosseus nerve injury following elbow arthroscopy. Arthroscopy 13:756–758
22. Gay DM, Raphael BS, Weiland AJ (2010) Revision arthroscopic contracture release in the elbow resulting in an ulnar nerve transection: a case report. J Bone Joint Surg Am 92:1246–1249
23. Sahajpal D, Blonna D, O'Driscoll S (2010) Anteromedial elbow arthroscopy portals in patients with prior ulnar nerve transposition or subluxation. Arthroscopy 26(8):1045–1052
24. Dumonski ML, Arciero RA, Mazzocca AD (2006) Ulnar nerve palsy after elbow arthroscopy. Arthroscopy 22(5):577 e1–3
25. Hahn M, Grossman JA (1998) Ulnar nerve laceration as a result of elbow arthroscopy. J Hand Surg Br 23:109
26. Reddy AS, Kvitne RS, Yocum LA, Elattrache NS, Glousman RE, Jobe FW (2000) Arthroscopy of the elbow: a long-term clinical review. Arthroscopy 16(6):588–594
27. Kovachevich R, Steinmann S (2012) Arthroscopic ulnar nerve decompression in the setting of elbow osteoarthritis. J Hand Surg 37A:663–668
28. Savoie FH 3rd (2007) Guidelines to becoming an expert elbow arthroscopist. Arthroscopy 23(11):1237–1240
29. Haapaniemi T, Berggren M, Adolfsson L (1999) Complete transaction of the median and radial nerves during arthroscopic release of post-traumatic elbow contracture. Arthroscopy 15:784–787

30. Adams JE, Merten SM, Steinmann SP (2007) Arthroscopic-assisted treatment of coronoid fractures. Arthroscopy 23:1060–1065
31. Adams JE, Wolff LH III, Merten SM, Steinmann SP (2008) Osteoarthritis of the elbow: results of arthroscopic osteophyte resection and capsulectomy. J Shoulder Elbow Surg 17:126–131
32. Gofton W, King G (2001) Heterotopic ossification following elbow arthroscopy. Arthroscopy 17:E2
33. Hughes SC, Hildebrand KA (2010) Heterotopic ossification—a complication of elbow arthroscopy: a case report. J Shoulder Elbow Surg 19:e1–e5
34. Sodha S, Nagda SH, Sennett BJ (2006) Heterotopic ossification in a throwing athlete after elbow arthroscopy. Arthroscopy 22:802.e1–802.e3
35. Ball CM, Meunier M, Galatz LM, Calfee R, Yamaguchi K (2002) Arthroscopic treatment of post-traumatic elbow contracture. J Shoulder Elbow Surg 11:624–629
36. Krishnan SG, Harkins DC, Pennington SD, Harrison DK, Burkhead WZ (2007) Arthroscopic ulnohumeral arthroplasty for degenerative arthritis of the elbow in patients under fifty years of age. J Shoulder Elbow Surg 16:443–448
37. Redden JF, Stanley D (1993) Arthroscopic fenestration of the olecranon fossa in the treatment of osteoarthritis of the elbow. Arthroscopy 9:14–16
38. Rubenthaler F, Wiese M, Senge A, Keller L, Wittenberg RH (2005) Long-term follow-up of open and endoscopic Hohmann procedures for lateral epicondylitis. Arthroscopy 21:684–690
39. Clasper JC, Carr AJ (2001) Arthroscopy of the elbow for loose bodies. Ann R Coll Surg Engl 83:34–36
40. Baumgarten TE, Andrews JR, Satterwhite YE (1998) The arthroscopic classification and treatment of osteochondritis dissecans of the capitellum. Am J Sports Med 26:520–523
41. Feldman MD (1997) Arthroscopic excision of type II capitellar fractures. Arthroscopy 13:743–748
42. McLaughlin RE II, Savoie FH III, Field LD, Ramsey JR (2006) Arthroscopic treatment of the arthritic elbow due to primary radiocapitellar arthritis. Arthroscopy 22:63–69
43. Timmerman LA, Andrews JR (1994) Arthroscopic treatment of posttraumatic elbow pain and stiffness. Am J Sports Med 22:230–235
44. Phillips BB, Strasburger S (1998) Arthroscopic treatment of arthrofibrosis of the elbow joint. Arthroscopy 14:38–44
45. Dexel J, Schneiders W, Kasten P (2011) Subcutaneous emphysema of the upper extremity after elbow arthroscopy. Arthroscopy 27(7):1014–1017

Elbow Arthroscopy: The Future

10

Felix Savoie III and Michael J. O'Brien

Elbow arthroscopy has made great advances since the Andrews and Carson article in 1985 [1]. Early limited indications of diagnostic arthroscopy and removal of loose bodies have expanded to include debridement of conditions such as arthritis, synovitis, and epicondylitis. As surgeons have gained familiarity with the elbow joint, instrumentation and techniques have improved. Experience gained during residency programs and fellowships is providing earlier training in arthroscopic procedures, and surgeons are emerging from training programs as experienced arthroscopists. Procedures once reserved for open cases, such as repairs of fractures and ligamentous injuries, are now being performed arthroscopically with increasing frequency. The future of elbow arthroscopy will likely continue to grow, as we do not yet know the bounds of its use. The future may include uses in arthroscopic interposition arthroplasty and prosthetic arthroplasty, as well as repairs on the medial side of the elbow.

This chapter aims to highlight current advanced arthroscopic techniques in the elbow, as well as possible future procedures on the horizon. As with most orthopaedic conditions, the indications for surgery are pain and functional impairment despite appropriate non-operative treatment. Certain acute injuries will require acute repair. The arthroscopic techniques and post-operative rehabilitation will be presented in each section.

F. Savoie III (✉) · M. J. O'Brien
Tulane University School of Medicine, 1430 Tulane Avenue, SL32,
New Orleans, LA 70112, USA
e-mail: fsavoie@tulane.edu; ritarichardson08@gmail.com

M. J. O'Brien
e-mail: mobrien@tulane.edu

L. A. Pederzini (ed.), *Elbow Arthroscopy*,
DOI: 10.1007/978-3-642-38103-4_10, © ISAKOS 2013

10.1   Arthroscopic Triceps Tendon Repair

Triceps tendon ruptures are increasingly more common as our aging patient population attempts to maintain an active lifestyle. Once a rare injury seen mostly in bodybuilders, it is now seen with increasing frequency. The triceps takes its name from the three heads which originate from the humerus and infraglenoid tubercle of the scapula. It inserts in a fan-like fashion on the posterior aspect of the olecranon and proximal ulna. Injuries of the triceps may take the form of partial or complete avulsion from the bone, intra substance muscle tears, or tears at the muscle-tendon junction.

Most patients with this injury will experience pain or a "pop" with press-type activities. This may occur during push-ups, chest press, or most commonly during bench press, when the weight-lifter loses control of the bar. Partial tears may begin with these activities, as well as during dips or overhead triceps extensions. Physical examination begins with observation for swelling and ecchymosis posterior in the elbow. A palpable gap in the extensor mechanism can often be detected in both partial and complete tears. Patients with complete tears may have a complete loss of the ability to extend the elbow against gravity, whereas those with partial or degenerative tears may retain elbow extension in a weakened, painful state. In patients with subtle tears, trying to extend the elbow from a fully flexed position reproduces pain directly over the site of the injury (i.e. triceps stress test).

Radiographs may show a small avulsion fracture off the tip of the olecranon. Diagnosis can be confirmed with magnetic resonance imaging (MRI), which may be helpful in cases of partial tears.

An arthroscopic triceps repair has previously been described by Savoie et al. [2]. The patient is placed in the prone or lateral decubitus position. Care is taken to palpate the ulnar nerve, and assure that it does not subluxate out of its groove. The initial portal is a proximal anterior medial or proximal anterior lateral portal for diagnostic arthroscopy of the anterior compartment. Many patients with this injury are very active and may be avid weightlifters. Pathology in the anterior compartment may include loose bodies or small osteophytes on the tip of the coronoid. This can be addressed before proceeding to the posterior compartment.

The initial posterior portal is a posterior central portal, located approximately 3 cm proximal to the tip of the olecranon. Care must be taken not to stray medial to midline for all posterior portals, for risk of damage to the ulnar nerve. Normally a trans-tendon portal, in most triceps avulsions this portal actually goes through the tear. Next, a posterior lateral portal is established along the lateral border of the triceps tendon. The torn triceps tendon is visualized. The arthroscope is moved to the posterior lateral portal, and the shaver is placed in the posterior central portal. The tip of the olecranon is debrided through this portal, as is the torn edge of the tendon (Fig. 10.1a–d). A central olecranon bursa portal is then established, and a double-loaded suture anchor is inserted into the tip of the olecranon. The anchor is angled toward the coronoid to avoid inadvertent penetration of the articular surface.

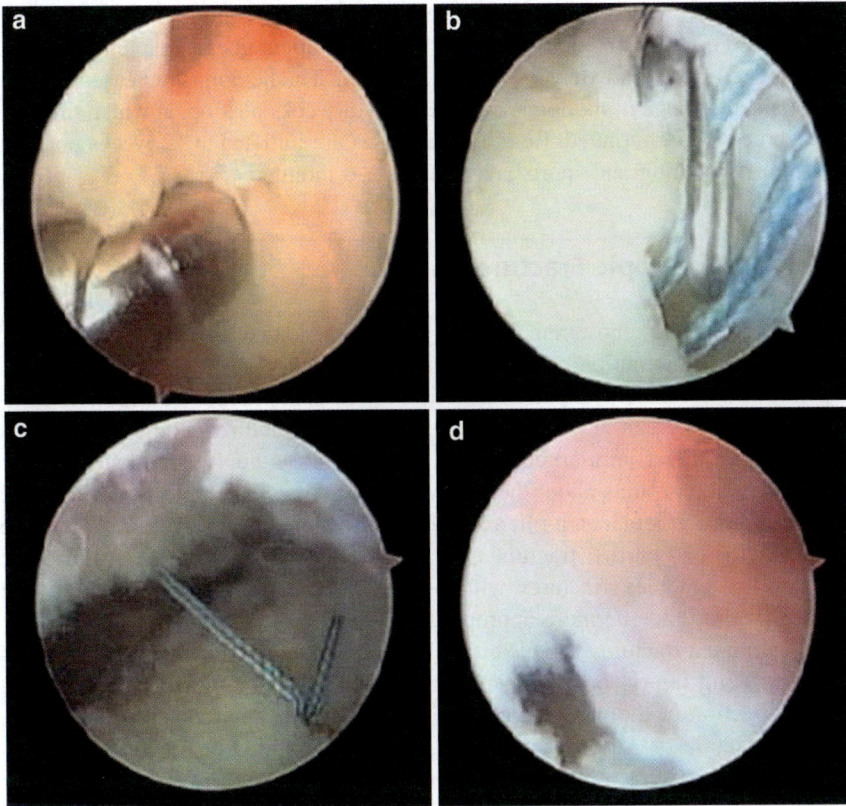

Fig. 10.1 Arthroscopic triceps repair. **a** The arthroscope and the shaver in the posterior compartment, debriding the torn edge of the triceps tendon. **b** The suture anchor is placed in the tip of the olecranon with suture shuttle retrieving suture. **c** A mattress suture has been placed in the torn triceps tendon. **d** The mattress suture has been tied subcutaneously, securing the triceps to the tip of the olecranon and sealing the joint

A retrograde suture retriever is placed percutaneously though the medial and lateral aspects of the proximal triceps tendon, retrieving the sutures from the anchor. Two mattress sutures are usually required to capture the tendon and complete the proximal part of the repair. After subcutaneous retrieval, they are tied with a sliding knot. This secures the proximal part of the tendon to the tip of the olecranon and seals the joint. The arthroscope is then placed directly into the olecranon bursa portal. The previous sutures can be left long and retrieved through the bursa portal. Crossing the sutures and incorporating them into a second knotless suture anchor more distal down the ulna creates a suture bridge construct that compresses the tendon down to the bone. In similar fashion, the first sutures can be cut, a second anchor placed more distally in the ulna, and the distal end of the triceps tendon can be tied down with simple sutures through the second anchor [3].

Post-operatively, the patient is placed into an anterior splint with the elbow in full extension. At the first post-operative visit, the patient goes into a hinged elbow brace, locked from full extension to 30° of flexion. The flexion is increased 10° per week until full range of motion is obtained at 6–8 weeks post-op, at which time the elbow brace is discontinued. Resistive exercises are initiated at 12 weeks post-op, with return to lifting and sports activities at 4–6 months.

10.2 Arthroscopic Fracture Repair

Fractures about the elbow remain a very common injury. Fractures can be very daunting, as comminution can distort the normal anatomy, major neurovascular structures are in close proximity to the joint, and post-operative stiffness is common. Arthroscopy can aid with fracture management and reduction, as it affords the surgeon a direct intra-articular view of the joint without disrupting the static and dynamic constraints about the elbow. This facilitates the reduction, limits the amount of intra-articular step-off, and avoids iatrogenic instability. Simple fracture patterns with one or two fracture fragments are very amenable to arthroscopic fixation. For complex fractures with severe comminution, open reduction and internal fixation may be more appropriate.

As with most fractures, the history will often include a traumatic injury such as a fall, sporting injury, or motor vehicle accident. The examination begins with close inspection of the involved extremity, looking for open wounds or punctate bleeding. Gentle palpation can localize pain, and crepitus of fracture fragments may be present. Gentle range of motion may reveal a block to forearm rotation or elbow flexion and extension. Pain and apprehension will likely limit the exam. Care must be taken to perform a careful neurologic examination in the case of any fracture or dislocation. The shoulder and wrist should routinely be examined. Routine radiographs of the elbow will diagnose most fractures. Computed tomography (CT) scan may be helpful to identify fracture fragments when severe comminution is present.

Simple fractures such as condylar fractures with one fracture line, capitellar shear fractures, radial head fractures with one or two fragments, and large coronoid fractures can be managed very well arthroscopically. Initially the arthroscope is usually placed in a proximal anterior medial portal to allow visualization of the lateral structures. Upon entrance into the elbow joint, abundant hematoma is encountered. A shaver placed in a proximal anterior lateral portal can be used to evacuate this hematoma and visualize the fracture line. During the initial debridement, limited use of suction is advised, as tearing in the capsule and overlying brachialis may place the radial nerve in close proximity. The tip of the shaver may be used like a probe to manipulate the fracture fragments.

For radial head fractures (Fig. 10.2a–b) and capitellar shear fractures (Fig. 10.3a–b), a Freer elevator introduced through an anterior lateral portal at the level of the radio capitellar joint can manipulate fracture fragments. Using

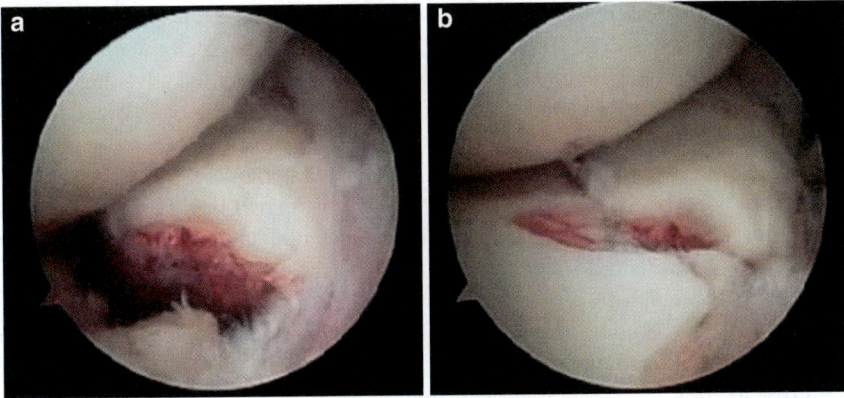

Fig. 10.2 Radial head fracture. A Mason Type II radial head fracture viewed from the proximal anterior medial portal before reduction (**a**) and after internal fixation with a headless compression screw (**b**)

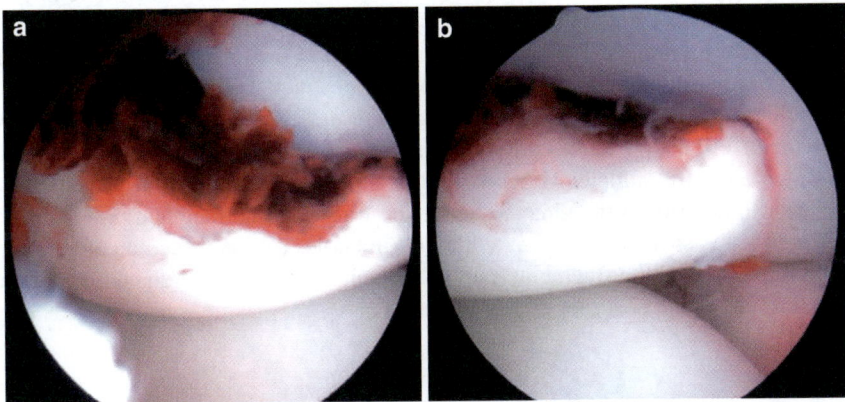

Fig. 10.3 Capitellar shear fracture. A Type I capitellar fracture (coronal shear fracture or Hahn-Steinthal fragment) viewed from the proximal anterior medial portal before reduction (**a**) and after internal fixation with headless compression screws (**b**)

arthroscopic instruments, the fracture is reduced, and provisional fixation with Kirschner wires can hold the reduction. Fluoroscopic images confirm reduction and pin placement. Headless cannulated screws can be placed over the pins for definitive fixation, from lateral to medial for radial head fractures and from posterior to anterior for capitellum fractures. The headless screws avoid articular cartilage erosion or impingement during elbow range of motion.

Rolla et al. [4] reported preliminary results for six patients who underwent arthroscopic reduction and internal fixation for radial head fractures. All patients returned to their pre-injury level of function within 6 months. Michels et al. [5]

presented 5 year follow-up data on 14 patients treated with an arthroscopic technique for Mason Type II radial head fractures. The mayo elbow performance (MEP) scores were excellent in 11 and good in three. A potential advantage of this arthroscopic technique was the observation that a single screw was usually sufficient to obtain stability.

In the case of condylar fractures of the distal humerus (Fig. 10.4a–b), the fracture line can be manipulated with the tip of the shaver or a Freer elevator. A large bone reduction clamp can be placed on the medial and lateral epicondyles to reduce the fracture and hold compression across the fracture site. Direct visualization with the scope in the anterior compartment can minimize step-off of the articular cartilage. Guide pins can be placed under fluoroscopic guidance from lateral to medial, and internal fixation performed with cannulated screws for definitive fixation. The reduction clamp should be left in place during drilling and screw placement; removing the clamp during either step could result in loss of reduction and fracture displacement.

Operative intervention for coronoid process fractures is recommended for Regan and Morrey [6] Type III fractures and any fracture that interferes with joint motion. When comminution precludes fixation, loose debris can be removed arthroscopically. Larger coronoid fractures can be treated effectively with arthroscopic techniques. The arthroscope is placed in the proximal anterior lateral portal to view the medial side of the elbow. The fracture fragments are reduced and held with a tibial anterior cruciate ligament drill guide. A guide pin can then be drilled from the posterior cortex of the ulna to engage the fracture fragment. If the fragment is of sufficient size, a single cannulated screw can be placed from posterior to anterior in the ulna to engage the fragment and maintain reduction. If the fragment is small or comminuted, two drills holes can be placed on either side of the fracture, and the fragments can be lassoed with a free suture and tied over a bone bridge on the posterior cortex of the ulna.

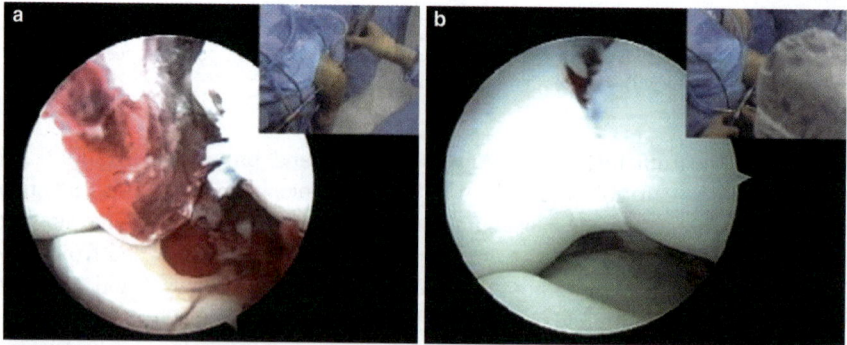

Fig. 10.4 Unicondylar Distal Humerus Fracture. A unicondylar distal humerus fracture with a single sagittal split before reduction (**a**) and after internal fixation with cannulated compression screws (**b**)

Adams et al. reported their experience with arthroscopically assisted reduction and fixation with four Type II and three Type III coronoid fractures [7]. Cannulated screw fixation was achieved antegrade over pins placed with the use of an anterior cruciate ligament guide. All five of the patients available for follow-up at an average of 2 years and 8 months had MEP scores of 100 %.

10.3 Endoscopic Biceps Repair

Tears of the distal biceps brachii tendon usually occur during forceful activity and produce a memorable event. The diagnosis is made clinically with history and physical exam. The tear occurs during eccentric contraction of the biceps muscle, such as lifting a heavy object or moving furniture. The patient will report feeling a "pop", immediate searing pain in the antecubital fossa and forearm, and developing ecchymosis over the ensuing several days. Typically, the pain markedly improves after several days. Inspection of the involved extremity will reveal ecchymosis in the antecubital fossa. A noticeable defect with proximal migration of the biceps muscle belly may or may not be noticeable, as the torn tendon may still be held in position by the lacertus fibrosus. Palpation of the anterior elbow from lateral to medial may reveal absence of the distal biceps tendon, producing a positive hook test. Range of motion will often be normal. Strength testing will often reveal deficits in resisted supination when compared to the contralateral extremity. The diagnosis is confirmed on MRI. Placing the arm in the *flexed abducted supinated* (FABS) position, as described by Giuffre and Moss, allows full-length views of the biceps brachii tendon from the musculotendinous junction to its insertion on the radial tuberosity in one or two sections [8].

Endoscopic investigation of the distal biceps tendon attachment provides dynamic assessment of the partially torn tendon through a range of motion. Viewing of the tendon through the insufflated bicipitoradial bursa provides a clear magnified view of the pathology by means of a minimally invasive procedure (Bain et al., Eames and Bain) [9, 10].

Endoscopy of the bicipitoradial bursa is performed with the patient under general anesthesia with the arm in the extended supinated position. A 2.5 cm longitudinal incision is made over the palpable biceps tendon 2 cm distal to the elbow crease. The lateral cutaneous nerve of the forearm is identified and protected. The distal biceps tendon and its bursa are identified with blunt finger dissection. The bursa is insufflated with 7–10 mL of normal saline. A small entry point is made on the radial side of the bursa at the apex for the arthroscope. The tendons are identifiable in this field of view and can be followed distally to the insertion on the radial tuberosity. The tendons can be viewed dynamically with forearm rotation or with traction applied to the biceps tendon. Careful inspection of the tendon can determine the extent, or percentage, of tendon damage. Tears involving less than 50 % of the tendon can be debrided with a motorized shaver through the same portal. A full-radius shaver without suction should be utilized.

Tears involving greater than 50 % of the tendon can be completed and repaired. A hooked electrocautery probe can complete the tear. The incision can then be extended to perform an open repair through a small incision with an endobutton, interference screw, or suture anchors into the radial tuberosity.

Sharma and MacKay [3] described an endoscopic technique for repair of complete tears using an endobutton technique. A 1.5 cm longitudinal incision is made in the midline of the anterior aspect of the arm at a point 5 cm proximal to the transverse anterior elbow crease. The ruptured end of the distal biceps tendon is delivered out of the wound. The ruptured end of the tendon is freshened and sutured to a fixed-loop endobutton. The endoscope is then placed down the tract of the distal biceps tendon and followed to its base, where the radial tuberosity can clearly be seen. The camera is removed, leaving the endoscope sheath in situ and positioned against the radial tuberosity. The sheath acts as a tissue protector for the surrounding neurovascular structures while the guide wire and reamers for the endobutton system are employed. A guide wire is placed bicortically, exiting the skin on the dorsal forearm. The endobutton reamer reams bicortically over the guide wire, followed by a 6 mm acorn reamer to ream only the near cortex. The sutures of the endobutton are loaded into the guide wire, and the guide wire is pulled out the dorsal aspect of the forearm. The endobutton is then "flipped" and can toggle on the dorsal aspect of the radius. Button position is confirmed with fluoroscopic images, and the biceps insertion site can be viewed directly with the arthroscope.

Post-operatively, range of motion is begun early. For tendon debridement, immediate range of motion is initiated, and full activities with resistive exercises can resume at 3–4 weeks. For tendon repair, immediate range of motion is initiated, with light activities begun at 4–6 weeks. Strengthening can begin at 12 weeks post-op.

10.4   Lateral Collateral Ligament Repair

Injury to the lateral collateral ligamentous complex of the elbow can cause severe dysfunction with activities of daily living. Unlike damage to the medial ulnar collateral ligament, with pain and instability only exacerbated by athletic activities, insufficiency of the radial ulnohumeral ligament (RUHL) makes even the most mundane activities difficult. Pushing up from a chair, shaking hands, or opening a door can cause pain and instability. The recognition and treatment of posterolateral rotatory instability (PLRI) of the elbow has grown since the original description by O'Driscoll et al. [11]. Late recognition requires open reconstruction with a graft. However, in the early setting, or after an acute injury, arthroscopic repair is possible.

Patients will complain of lateral sided elbow pain and popping with activities. They often report feeling a "clunk" or a "pop" when pushing off a surface or arising from a chair. This sensation can be reproduced on physical exam by asking the patient to push up from a chair with the hands fully supinated on the armrests (i.e. chair test). Lateral instability may best be demonstrated clinically with the pivot shift test of the elbow. First described O'Driscoll et al. [11], this test performed in the supine position may elicit gross instability or pain and apprehension.

Diagnostic imaging begins with routine radiographs. Radiographs may reveal an avulsion off of the posterior humeral lateral epicondyle in acute cases. Stress radiographs or fluoroscopic images while performing a pivot shift test may show the radial head and proximal ulna moving together in a subluxated and posterolaterally rotated position. MRI of the elbow can identify a lesion in the RUHL, especially with the addition of intra-articular contrast.

The surgical treatment of posterolateral instability may be divided into distinct subgroups based on cause: acute dislocations, recurrent dislocations, and PLRI. The procedures used may also be divided into subgroups based on available tissue at the time of reconstruction: repair of ligamentous avulsion, plications of the RUHL complex with or without repair to bone, and tendon graft reconstruction.

The anatomic injury pattern associated with acute and recurrent dislocations is avulsion of the RUHL, usually off the humeral attachment. Dislocations usually respond to non-operative management. The most common complication of non-operative management of acutely dislocated elbows is stiffness, not recurrent instability. However, several subsets of patients may benefit from operative intervention: patients with a humeral avulsion fracture seen on radiographs, patients requiring a high level of function, professional athletes, those with damage to multiple areas of the joint, and those with recurrent instability who have failed non-operative management of an elbow dislocation. These patients may be candidates for an arthroscopic repair of the RUHL (Fig. 10.5a–d).

The procedure begins with establishment of a proximal anterior medial portal for the arthroscope, and diagnostic arthroscopy of the anterior compartment. Abundant hematoma will be encountered in the acute setting, and may be removed with a shaver from a proximal anterior lateral portal. Tears in the anterior capsule and brachialis will be identified. Associated fractures of the coronoid, radial head, and distal humerus may also be encountered. The annular ligament should be inspected for laxity as it courses around the radial head. The forearm can be rotated to perform an arthroscopic evaluation of posterolateral rotatory instability as the forearm fully supinates.

The arthroscope is placed in the posterior central portal, 3 cm proximal to the tip of the olecranon. Hematoma in the posterior compartment can be evacuated with a shaver placed in the proximal posterolateral portal. The medial gutter is evaluated for tears in the capsule as well as loose bodies. Then the arthroscope is advanced down the posterolateral gutter. The lateral gutter is debrided and cleared of hematoma, taking care to remain close to the ulna and avoid damage to the torn RUHL. The posterior distal humerus is also lightly debrided, and site of the avulsion of the RUHL localized. It is usually directly lateral and slightly inferior to the center of the olecranon fossa. A bare area can be easily identified at the site of the ligament avulsion.

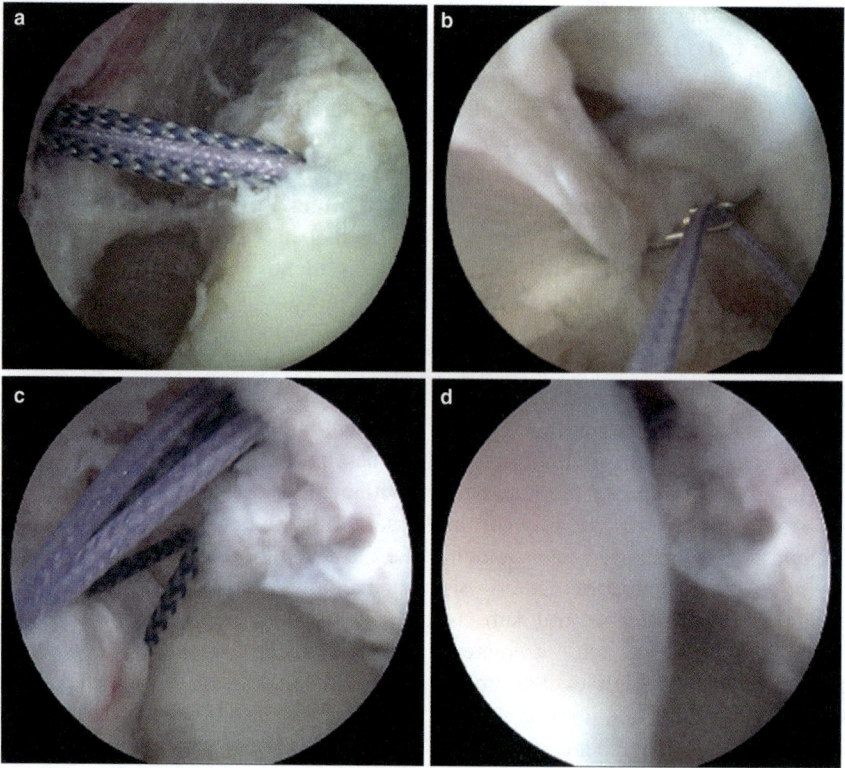

Fig. 10.5 Arthroscopic RUHL repair. **a** Suture anchor placement in the posterior humeral lateral epicondyle is shown. **b** Suture is retrieved through the torn RUHL down the lateral gutter. **c** Placement of mattress sutures in the torn RUHL is shown. **d** After tying the mattress sutures, the arthroscope is effectively pushed out of the lateral gutter as the gutter is closed down

After the avulsion site has been identified and debrided, a double-loaded suture anchor may be placed into the humerus at the origin of the RUHL. One suture at a time, the sutures are placed down the lateral gutter and retrieved to place two horizontal mattress sutures through the non-injured part of the ligament. In the setting of a bony avulsion, one set is placed around the fracture fragment and the other set distal to the fracture fragment. The sutures are tensioned with the arthroscope viewing from the lateral gutter, which should have the effect of pushing the arthroscope out of the gutter. The elbow is extended, the sutures retrieved, and the sutures are tied beneath the anconeus muscle. The ligament is lax with extension and tightens with flexion. Therefore, we recommend placing the elbow in pronation and 45–60° of flexion during tensioning to prevent over-tightening and the resultant loss of flexion.

Post-operatively, patients are placed into a posterior splint with the elbow flexed to 30°. Fluoroscopic images can confirm reduction in the splint, and the elbow can be further flexed as needed to maintain reduction. At the first post-op visit after 5–7 days, the splint is removed and the patient is placed into a hinged elbow brace that allows comfortable movement from 0 to 45° of flexion. The hinged elbow brace is discontinued at 6–8 weeks post-op, at which time full range of motion should be restored, and more aggressive exercises and strengthening can progress with physical therapy.

10.5   Bone Grafting for Osteochondritis Dissecans

Osteochondritis dissecans (OCD) is a challenging condition for the treating orthopaedic surgeon. It is common in young athletes, especially baseball players and gymnasts. The disease can cause significant pain in the young athlete, with inability to load the arm or fully extend the elbow. The pain and dysfunction often limits participation in sports.

The patient will complain of lateral sided pain in the elbow. Elbow stiffness, with loss of terminal extension, is a common finding. Mechanical symptoms of popping, catching, or grinding may be present, and may signal the treating physician to the presence of possible intra-articular loose bodies. On examination, swelling in the lateral gutter may be present. The posterolateral elbow will be tender to palpation, with point tenderness over the posterior capitellum with the elbow flexed to 90°. Range of motion will be limited when compared to the contralateral extremity, with a loss of 10–20° of terminal extension. Patients may have a positive grind test, with reproducible pain and mechanical symptom with axial load, valgus stress, and forearm rotation. This loads the radiocapitellar joint and pain is reproduced as the radial head contacts the lesion in the capitellum. Radiographs may show the lesion, and the diagnosis is confirmed with MRI. MRI arthrogram may be particularly helpful in investigating the status of the cartilage cap. If there is separation or dislodgment of the cartilage cap, contrast dye will infiltrate along the defect in the cartilage, showing the amount of displacement.

Surgery is indicated for continued pain and dysfunction after appropriate non-operative treatment has failed to provide relief. Surgery is also indicated when loose bodies are present, causing mechanical symptoms in the joint. Initial surgical management includes arthroscopic debridement of lesions and either fixation of chondral fragments, or removal of fragments followed by drilling of the base of the lesion.

OCD lesions with bone loss become a difficult problem to treat. Significant bone loss can preclude simple drilling of the lesion. Loss of the lateral aspect of the capitellum, or "shoulder" of the capitellum, can lead to containment problems and possible instability. Bone loss can be diagnosed on standard radiographs, and the amount of bone loss can be further quantified by advanced imaging with CT or MRI. Bone grafting of the defect may become necessary, and this can be performed arthroscopically.

After diagnostic arthroscopy in the anterior compartment to remove loose bodies and debride synovitis, the main portion of the procedure is performed in the posterior compartment. The arthroscope is placed in a posterior lateral portal, and advanced down the lateral gutter. Keeping the in-flow in the anterior compartment through a proximal anterior medial portal can help water flow retrograde up the lateral gutter and keep the lateral gutter expanded to enhance visualization. A 70° scope facilitates looking forward upon the capitellum to fully view the defect. Establishment of both a standard and an additional distal soft-spot portal on the posterior lateral aspect of the elbow allows instrumentation to access the OCD lesion. Increasing flexion past 90° brings the entire capitellum into view, and the two portals facilitate advanced surgery without damaging the radial head. A shaver can debride the defect, removing soft tissue debris or bony loose bodies. Once significant bone loss is confirmed, the decision is made to proceed with arthroscopic bone grafting. Several options exist for pre-contoured allograft cancellous bone plugs of varying diameter. The defect can be sized using standardized sizing templates. A bone plug 1–2 mm smaller than the size of the defect is chosen. Through the distal soft-spot portal, the correct angle can be determined. A trocar is used to remove a plug of bone from the central aspect of the defect. The allograft bone plug can then be inserted back into the capitellum, following the same angle. This bone plug can fill the defect, re-establishing the convexity of the capitellum. The bone plug can be left in situ in this position, or it can be covered with a biologic patch (Fig. 10.6a–c) or cartilage graft. (Figure 10.7a–b) shows a small posterolateral incision with a cartilage graft composed of live cartilage cells covering an allograft bone plug.

Post-operatively, the patient is placed in a hinged elbow brace for 6 weeks to off-load the lateral elbow. Early range of motion is initiated in the hinged elbow brace, while weight-bearing through the elbow is avoided. Strengthening and resistive exercises are initiated at 12 weeks. Return to play is permitted at 6 months. Repeat MRI can be obtained at 6 months to confirm incorporation of the grafts into the capitellum.

10.6 Arthroscopically Assisted Arthroplasty

Arthritis of the elbow joint can be a very debilitating condition, especially when it occurs in young adults. Osteoarthritis often causes a painless loss of motion, with crepitus caused by osteophytes and possible loose bodies. On the contrary, post-traumatic arthritis can be a painful condition with resulting stiffness and loss of motion.

When conservative measures fail to relieve symptoms of pain and stiffness, arthroscopic surgery may be an option. Ulno-humeral arthroplasty has long proved to have good results in eliminating mechanical symptoms, restoring motion, and alleviating pain. Creating a large drill hole communicating between the olecranon

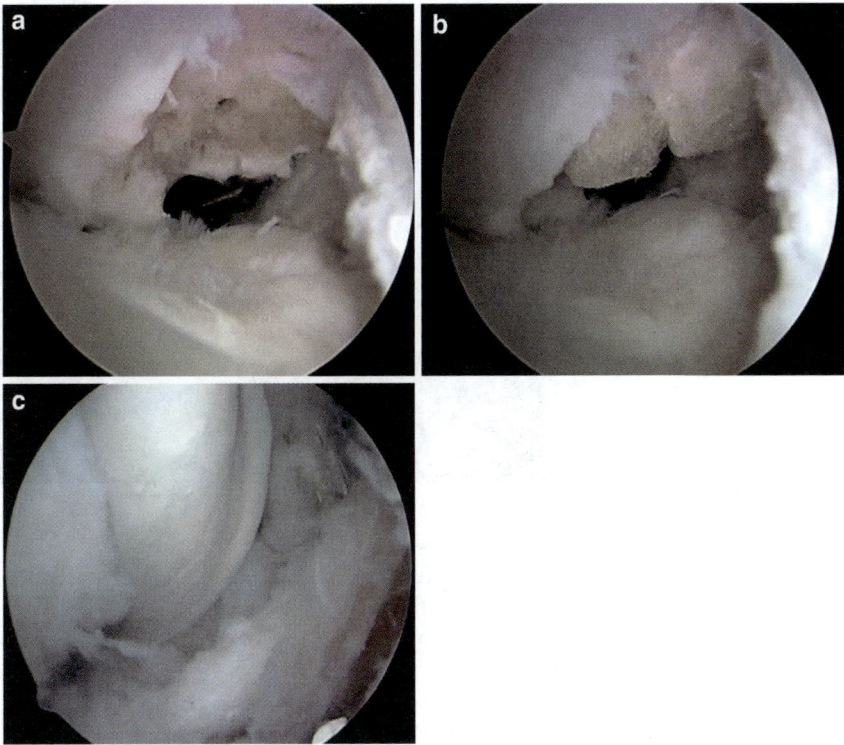

Fig. 10.6 Bone grafting for OCD. Osteochondritis dissecans of the capitellum with bone loss and loss of the lateral "shoulder" is viewed from the lateral gutter, after drilling of the lesion (**a**), after bone grafting with allograft plugs (**b**), and after biologic resurfacing (**c**)

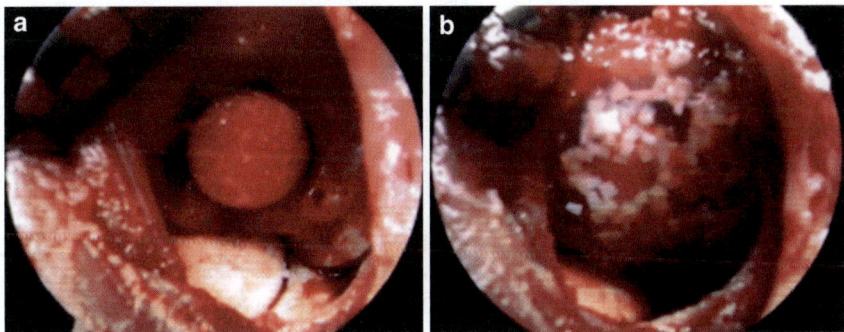

Fig. 10.7 Cartilage grafting for OCD. Osteochondritis dissecans of the capitellum is viewed through a small posterolateral incision, after bone grafting with allograft plugs (**a**), and after resurfacing with a live cartilage graft (**b**)

Fig. 10.8 Arthroscopic
biologic resurfacing of the
radiocapitellar joint is shown

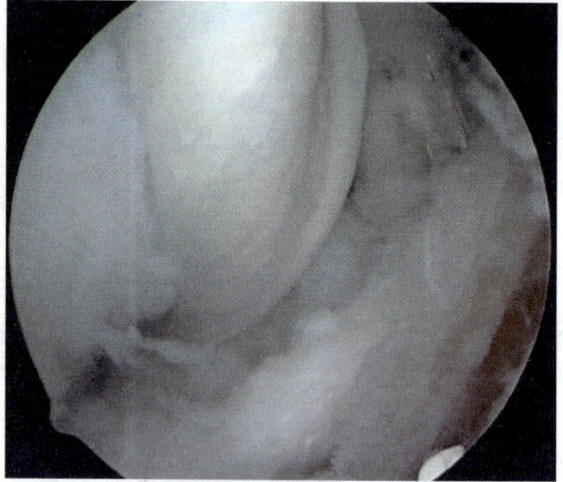

fossa and coronoid fossa vents the distal humerus, removing impinging osteophytes in the anterior and posterior compartments.

In the future, arthroscopic interposition arthroplasty or prosthetic arthroplasty
likely will become an option. Biologic resurfacing of the radiocapitellar joint
(Fig. 10.8) may be possible through cannula systems to insert biologic grafts into
the elbow joint. The graft may be secured by suturing into surrounding soft tissue
or with use of suture anchors. In a similar fashion, prosthetic replacement of the
radial head or capitellum may be accomplished by arthroscopic assistance through
small incisions using minimally invasive techniques.

10.7   Conclusions

The field of elbow arthroscopy has advanced greatly in the past 25 years. Innovative arthroscopists continue to expand indications and develop new surgical
techniques enlarging the boundaries of its use. Procedures such as fixation of
fractures and ligamentous avulsions are now being performed arthroscopically
with increasing frequency. It is not difficult to imagine that in the not so distant
future, additional surgeries will be performed with arthroscopic assistance, such as
arthroscopic interposition arthroplasty, prosthetic arthroplasty, and ligamentous
repairs on the medial side of the elbow. The creative and intelligent minds of
current arthroscopic surgeons will continue to push the envelope and develop new
operative techniques until elbow arthroscopy of the future becomes reality.

References

1. Andrews JR, Carson WG (1985) Arthroscopy of the elbow. Arthroscopy 1985(1):97–107
2. Savoie FH III, Field LD, O'Brien MJ (2010) Arthroscopic triceps repair. In: Savoie FH III, Field LD (ed) AANA advanced arthroscopy, the elbow and wrist.: Saunders Elsevier, Philadelphia: 132–135
3. Sharma S, MacKay G (2005) Endoscopic repair of distal biceps tendon using an endobutton. Arthroscopy 21:897
4. Rolla PR, Surace MF, Bini A, Pilato G (2006) Arthroscopic treatment of fractures of the radial head. Arthroscopy, 22:233 e1–233 e6
5. Michels F, Pouliart N, Handelberg F (2007) Arthroscopic management of mason type II radial head fractures. Knee Surg Sports Traumatol Arthrosc 15:1244–1250
6. Regan W, Morrey B (1989) Fractures of the coronoid process of the ulna. J Bone Joint Surg Am 71:1348–1354
7. Adams JE, Merton SM, Steinmann SP (2007) Arthroscopic-assisted treatment of coronoid fractures. Arthroscopy 2007(23):1060–1065
8. Giuffre BM, Moss MJ (2004) Optimal positioning for MRI of the distal biceps brachii tendon: flexed abducted supinated view. AJR Am J Roentgenol 182:944–946
9. Bain GI, Johnson JL, Turner PC (2008) Treatment of partial distal biceps tendon tears. Sports Med Arthrosc 16:154–161
10. Eames MHA, Bain GI (2006) Distal biceps tendon endoscopy and anterior elbow arthroscopy portal. Tech Shoulder Elbow Surg 7:139–142
11. O'Driscoll SW, Bell DF, Morrey BF (1991) Posterolateral rotatory instability of the elbow. J Bone Joint Surg Am 73:440–446